Ayurveda for Beginners

Understand & Apply Essential Ayurvedic Principles & Practices

By: Jane Rivers

Table of Contents

Table of Contents

Introduction

Understanding Ayurveda, or what might also be called "ayurvedic medicine," is a specified lifestyle system that people from India have used for more than five centuries. Ayurveda promotes good health practices by way of prevention and the treatment of illness and/or disease through multiple lifestyle practices, and by the express use of herbal remedies and dietary influences.

Ayurvedic medicine tries its best to be "holistic," which means incorporating the physical body, the spiritual body, and the mind functionality as a whole. And Ayurveda not only treats an individual's physical complaints, it also adapts lifestyle practices as preferences to help maintain and improve overall health.

Essential to Ayurveda are the 5 elements within nature. More specifically known as: space, air, fire, water, and earth which combine within the human body as 3 symbiotic integrations (vata, pitta, and kapha) known collectively as doshas. These doshas resemble the basic elements of nature and represent the specific functions within the human body's functioning. According to Ayurveda, a balance of these doshas is said to be required for the optimal health of an individual.

Air & Space = Vata

Vata is in control of muscle and joint movement, along with breathing, and the heartbeat. Additionally, vata controls an individual's anxiety, fear, pain, and other functions concerned with the nervous system of the physical body.

Fire & Water = Pitta

Pitta is said to control bodily functions including metabolism, digestion, intelligence, and skin color. Pitta is concerned with the emotions of anger, hate, and jealousy, too.

Earth & Water = Kapha

Kapha represents the physical structure of the body, as well as the immune system. Emotional responses are said to be controlled by kapha including calmness, forgiveness, love, and greediness.

Interestingly, the doshas are determined at the time of an individual's biological conception and are representative of an individual's physical makeup and their overall character or personality. A person with a 'vata' makeup tends to have a smaller, thinner build. The 'pitta' body type is more of a medium and muscular build. The 'kapha' look is usually bigger and quite well-developed. Most people are considered to have a combination of these doshas, with one type being most dominant overall.

Ayurvedic medicine believes that when an imbalance occurs in any of the three doshas, illness will result. Ayurvedic medicine heals sickness in many ways, including the utilization of herbal remedies, dietary inclusions or emissions, and via exercise and some other complementary modalities which will be discussed later. According to the ayurvedic philosophy, you can enhance the practice through the practice of yoga, by including meditation, and/or counselling as treatment options.

What Can Ayurveda Medicine Do for Humans?

Some people use it to maintain their overall health, as a stress reduction, to improve flexibility, to gain strength, and/or improve stamina. Practices like yoga and meditation can be helpful for people with diseases like arthritis, high blood pressure, and even asthma. Ayurveda also promotes a truer diet for maintaining good health and treating disease. Herbal medicines are prescribed based on an individual's dosha type.

Is Ayurveda Considered to Be a Safe Practice?

Ayurvedic practices such as a great diet and the inclusion of yoga and meditation are safe ways to promote an individual's health. Scientific studies reflect this, too. For a long-term illness, combining Ayurveda medicine with conventional medical treatment can work, however, many choose either one or the other, and a consultation with a trusted practitioner is always recommended.

Some 'Western' conformists do not believe that Ayurveda is completely safe, but its historical use dates much earlier than modern medicine. So, its efficacy may be argued either way, and opinions might differ, depending upon who is arguing, either for or against it.

Ayurvedic herbal doses can be like conventional medicines in that they may cause side effects, trigger allergic reactions, or perhaps even interact with other medicines or herbs being consumed. Some medicines may contain high levels of heavy metals which can be toxic or harmful to the human body. This is true for both Western and Eastern practices.

You should always speak with your trusted practioner about any complementary health practices or medicines, including herbal remedies that you'd like to try or are already using. Sometimes it's difficult to know whether or not some medicines go together, or if they're disagreeing by way of functionality within the body.

These next chapters will introduce you to Ayurvedic medicine, and aim to give you a simple, yet broader understanding of an Eastern system which has been utilized for centuries; borne from the heart of India.

Chapter 1: The Easy Way to Wellbeing Through Vital Ayurveda Principles

Ayurveda is considered by many scholars to be the oldest healing science around today. In Sanskrit, the word "Ayurveda" translates as "the science of life."

The understanding of Ayurvedic principles originated in ancient India and is often called the "mother of all healing." It is based upon the ancient Vedic culture and was handed down for many thousands of years in a particularly oral tradition from accomplished masters who taught it to their disciples. Some of this knowledge was printed a few thousand years ago, but unfortunately, much of it is unobtainable. The principles of many of the natural healing systems known in the West, such as *polarity* and *homeopathy,* have their basis in Ayurveda, .

Inner Balance & Your Constitution

Ayurveda places great importance on prevention rather than cure, and therefore encourages the bridge to health through close attention and adhesion to balance in an individual's life, including correct thinking, diet, lifestyle, and the use of herbs as medicinal foods, or foods as medicine.

Knowledge through Ayurveda enables individuals to understand how to create the unique and important balance of body, mind, and consciousness according to one's own individual makeup and choice to proceed with a regime, and how to make lifestyle changes to bring about and maintain this overall balance.

The Uniqueness of You & Ayurveda

Just as everyone has a unique DNA pattern, each person also has a particular pattern of energy, including the individual combination of physical, mental, and emotional characteristics. This unique constitution is determined at conception by various factors and remains the same throughout an individual's life.

Many factors, both internally and externally, act upon us to disturb the balance and are seen most usually as a change in one's constitution from the balanced state which we are supposed to sustain for the long term.

It's also true that the emotional and physical stresses make up an individual's emotional state, including the incorporations of diet and food choices, seasons and weather, physical or emotional trauma, and professional and family relationships.

Each factor can be understood, and the individual can take appropriate action to quash or minimize the effects, or eliminate the causes of imbalance to re-establish the original and balanced constitution.

The Natural Order is Balance

It's also true that balance *is* the natural "order," whereas imbalance is said to be "disorder." Great health is order; illness is disorder. It's also true that, according to Ayurveda, within the body there's a constant interaction between the

6

possibility of order and disorder. One who understands the nature and structure of disorder can then re-establish order. It's quite a profound knowing, in fact. It has spiritual backing, too. In the Chinese belief system, it's similar to the ying-yang understanding, which can be used here as a comparison of similarity.

The 3 Energies of the Physical Body

Ayurveda identifies 3 basic types of energy or principles of functionality that are present within everyone and in everything. Since there are no single words in English that convey such concepts, the original Sanskrit words are used. We have already mentioned these in the *Introduction;* vata, pitta, and kapha. These principles can be related to the basic biology of the human body.

True energy is required to create movement so that fluids (as well as nutrients) get to the cellular structures, therefore enabling the body to function at prime levels. Energy is also required to metabolize the nutrients within the cells and is necessary to lubricate and maintain the structure of the cells during their processes.

The Key 3 Ayurveda Principles

We have already had a brief discussion of these principles, but let's revisit them again so we can be more acquainted and learn them more easily.

Vata is the energy of movement.

Pitta is the energy of digestion or metabolism.

Kapha is the energy of lubrication and structure.

Every individual has the qualities of vata, pitta, and kapha, but one is usually primary, one secondary, and the third is usually least dominant of all. The cause of disease in Ayurveda is viewed as a lack of proper cellular function, due to either the excess or deficiency of vata, pitta, or kapha. Disease can also be caused by the presence of toxins within the body This is important and a key understanding because many individuals don't realize the toxicity within their own bodies. Toxins can be present within the foods, medications, in allergens (like pet fur), in water sources, within the air, within the atmosphere, in fabrics or paints, and in chemicals or sprays found within a home, business, region, or locality.

In Ayurveda, the body, the mind, and the consciousness, all work together to maintain the right balance. They are easily and effectively viewed as different facets of an individual's beingness that makes up the whole person.

The 5 Great Elements

To learn how to balance the body, the mind, and the consciousness, requires an understanding of how vata, pitta, and kapha work, and that they do so in combination with one another. Interestingly, according to Ayurvedic philosophy the whole cosmos is an interplay of the energies of the 5 great elements. As we already know, these are: space, air, fire, water, and earth.

The principles of vata, pitta, and kapha are combinations and extensions of these 5 elements which manifest as patterns that are said to be present in all of creation. In the physical body, vata is the subtle energy of movement, pitta is the energy of digestion and metabolism, and kapha is the energy that forms the body's structure and its lubrication. We'll take a look at the 3 principles a little more in depth now.

Vata: The Subtle Energy Concerning Movement

This principle is composed of the elements *space* and *air*.

It takes care of breathing, blinking, muscle and tissue movement, the pulsation of the heart, and every set of movements within the cytoplasm of the cells, including the cell membranes. When in order (or balance), vata allows creativity and flexibility. In disorder (or imbalance) vata allows fear and anxiety to take hold.

Pitta: The Expression of the Body's Metabolic System

This principle is composed of the elements *fire* and *water*.

It takes care of digestion, absorption, assimilation, nutrition, metabolism, and physical body temperature. When in order (or balance), pitta allows understanding and intelligence. Out of order (or imbalance), pitta allows anger, hatred, narcissism, and jealousy.

Kapha: The Thorough Energy Which Forms the Body's Structure

This principle is composed of the elements *earth* and *water*.

It takes care of the bones, muscles, and the tendons. It holds everything together. In fact, kapha supplies the water for all body parts and systems. It proceeds to lubricate the joints, moisturize the skin, and maintain overall immunity within the physical body. When in order (or balance), kapha allows love, calmness, peace, and forgiveness. Out of order (or imbalance), it allows attachment, greed, and envy.

Maintaining Balance Takes Careful Consideration

To maintain balance and to promote health, it is important to pay attention to all decisions related to an individual's wellbeing. Diet and lifestyle factors, which are appropriate to an individual constitution, will also strengthen the body, mind, and consciousness.

Ayurveda: The Complementary System of Healing

The basic difference between Ayurveda and Western medicine is important to understand. Western medicine generally focuses upon symptomatology and disease, and mostly uses drugs and surgery to rid the body of pathogens or diseased tissue. It's true that many lives have been saved by this fixing approach. In some instances, surgery is encouraged by Ayurveda. However, drug reliance, because of the toxicity involved, often weakens the body.

Ayurveda does not focus on the existence of disease. In fact, Ayurveda maintains that all life must be supported by energy which is in balance or "order." When there's minimal stress, and the flow of energy within a person is balanced or ordered, the body's natural defense systems will be strong enough to defend against disease.

It must be mentioned here that Ayurveda is not a substitute for Western medicine. Always seek a practitioner's advice and do your own research with regards to your choices. Ayurveda can, however, be used in conjunction with Western medicine.

We all have times when we don't feel ourselves, and we might even recognize that we're out of balance. Sometimes, we might have seen a practitioner only to be told that there's nothing truly wrong at all. According to Ayurveda philosophy, what's really occurring is that this imbalance has not yet become recognizable as a full-blown illness or disease. It is, however, serious enough to make the person notice some level of discomfort.

The Importance of Evaluation & the Treatment of Imbalances

Ayurveda encompasses various techniques for the assessment of an individual's health. The Ayurveda practitioner considers and evaluates key signs and symptoms of illness, especially with regards to the origin and cause of the first imbalance. They'll also consider the individual's suitability for various types of treatments.

After this, the Ayurveda practitioner will arrive at a diagnosis through efforts which include the use of direct questioning, careful observation, and a physical exam, including inference. Basic techniques like taking the pulse, observing the tongue, looking closely at the eyes and the body's form, and even listening to the tone of the voice are utilized during the overall assessment.

Some palliative and cleansing measures, when necessary, can be used to help eliminate any imbalance, along with suggestions for eliminating or managing the causes of the imbalance. Recommendations might be made up of the implementation of lifestyle changes, including starting and maintaining a suggested dietary inclusion, and the use of herbs. Sometimes, participating in a cleansing program, known as panchakarma, is suggested, and this is to help the body rid itself of accumulated toxins to gain more benefit from the various suggested measures of treatment, overall.

In essence, Ayurveda addresses all aspects of life. This includes the physical body, the mind, and the spirit, or consciousness of who we are. It understands that each of us is unique, and that each person responds differently to the many aspects which make up life, with each possessing different strengths and an array of weaknesses, too. Through insightful clarification, thorough understanding, and via experience, Ayurvedic medicine presents a true wealth of information on the relationships between their causes and effects, both immediately and subtlety, and for each individual.

Describing Vata

Vata provides the truest motion for all bodily processes and is extremely vital for health. Annually, vata is most prominent in the fall (autumn), and during the changeover of the seasons. Interestingly, these are the most important times to be careful with regards to diet and lifestyle factors. One main purpose of lifestyle considerations is to stabilize this motion. Having a planned-out routine is highly useful in assisting the predominantly vata individual to effectively ground all this moving energy.

A person who is vata dominant is blessed with a quick-witted mind, the ability to allow for flexibility, and is usually dominant with their own creativity. On a mental level, they usually grasp concepts very quickly too, but then forget them just as easily. Alert, restless, and fiercely active, vata people walk faster, talk more rapidly, and think faster, but are easily fatigued. They usually have less willpower, lack some confidence, impede their own boldness, and have a prevalence toward fluctuations in their character. This is when compared to other types. Quite often they'll feel unstable and ungrounded.

When unbalanced (or disordered), vata types may become fearful, nervous, and quite anxious. In the external world, vata types tend to earn money super quickly and spend it very quickly as well. They're generally not very good planners and may suffer from financial hardship because of this trait.

Vata types have an appetite and digestion process which can vary. They're usually attracted to foods like salad and raw vegetables, but their constitution is balanced by having warmer types, cooked foods, and sweet, sour, and salty tastes. With a tendency to produce less urine, their stools are often harder, dryer, and smaller in both size and quantity.

More specifically, vata resides in the colon as well as the brain, ears, bones, joints, thighs, and skin. Vata types are more prone to diseases involving the air principle, including emphysema, arthritis, pneumonia, or other airway issues such as asthma. Other common vata disorders include regular flatulence, tics, twitches, aching joints, dry hair, scaly skin, nerve disorders, constant constipation, and mental confusion. Vata in the physical body tends to increase with older age and is usually more obvious by the drying and wrinkling of the skin.

The major attributes of vata are light, cold, dry, rough, subtle, clear, and mobile. And any of these qualities in excess can cause a real disorder or imbalance. Frequent travel, especially by air, loud noises, overstimulation, drugs, sugar, and alcohol all create disorder for vata, as does overexposure to cold and colder liquids and foods.

Like the wind or air, vata types have a difficult time becoming grounded and maintaining this within their lives. Here, routine is difficult, but truly necessary if vata is to be lowered and controlled. It's really best for vata types to go to bed by 10 pm because they need more rest than the other types do. In general, people with dominant vata respond best to warm, slightly oily, moist, and heavier foods. Steam baths like saunas, humidifiers and moisture are helpful, too. A daily oil massage before hygiene care is also recommended.

Understanding Dietary Considerations

The simplest food guidelines for decreasing vata include warm and well-cooked foods. An individual should have smaller meals 3 or 4 times a day, and can snack as needed, while still maintaining a 2-hour gap between each smaller meal. Regularity for mealtimes is important for the dominant vata type. Great ideas can be soups, stews, and casseroles too. They can use more oil in cooking their foods than the other 2 dosha types and enjoy far better digestion if they limit their intake of raw foods.

While cooked vegetables are best for vata, the occasional salad with a good oily or creamy dressing is great. Foods such as tomatoes, potatoes, peppers, spinach, and eggplants should be avoided if the vata dominant has aching or stiff joints or muscles. Sweet, ripe, and juicy-type fruits are excellent for the dominant vata types. Additionally, dried fruits like raw apples and cranberries should be avoided. Fruit should always be eaten by itself and on an empty stomach.

Many vata types can satisfy their need for protein by the consistent use of dairy products, and they may also utilize eggs, chicken, fresh fish, turkey, and venison too. Legumes are difficult for this type to digest properly and should be consumed in minimal quantities by those trying to balance out vata. Additionally, legumes should be the split type and soaked very well before cooking. Cooking them with minimal oil and spices, like garlic, turmeric, cumin, coriander, and ginger will help prevent vata from becoming off balance or disordered.

It's also important to note that nuts and seeds are especially good for vata but are best used as butters or in milks. All dairy products are good for vata with harder cheeses needing to be eaten sparingly.

Additionally, spices are great, but should not be overused. Vatas can have about a half a glass of wine, diluted with water, either during or after a meal. Since vata people are prone to addiction, they should always avoid processed sugar, caffeine, and tobacco products. Utilizing relaxation and meditation to reduce vata is key.

To Balance Vata:

- Keep the individual warm
- Keep the individual calm
- Avoid cold, raw, or frozen foods
- Avoid extreme coldness
- Eat warmer foods and spices
- Keep a regular routine, always
- Get plenty of rest and relaxation

Describing Pitta

Pitta types have many of the attributes of fire. Fire is sharp, penetrating, hot, and agitating. And so, pitta people have warmer bodies, more penetrating ideas, and even a sharper intelligence. When out of balance, they can become very agitated and quick or short-tempered. The pitta body type is a medium height and build, with mixed or coppery-type skin. They might have many moles and freckles on their bodies, too. Their skin is warm and less wrinkled than the vata skin type. Their hair tends to be silkier and they often experience graying as a premature condition or even hair loss. Their eyes are medium in size and the conjunctiva is usually always moist. The nose is more pronounced, and the tip of the protrusion tends to be reddened somewhat.

It's also true that pitta-dominant types have a stronger metabolism, great digestion, and very strong appetites. They like plenty of food and liquids, and usually love hot spices and colder-type drinks. Here, their constitution is balanced by sweet, bitter, and the sour tastes. Pitta sleep is generally sound and of a medium duration. They produce large quantities of urine and feces, which can be yellowish in color, and soft and plentiful. They sweat easily and their hands and feet stay warm. Pitta people have a lower tolerance for sunlight, heat, and arduous physical work.

The mental capacity for pitta types are the characteristics of being alert and intelligent, and they have excellent powers of comprehension. However, they can be easily agitated and become aggressive, so might move toward hate, anger, and jealousy when disordered or imbalanced. In the external world, pitta types like to be leaders and planners, and they enjoy making moves towards material prosperity. They can enjoy showing off their wealth and possessions, too. Pitta people tend to have diseases involving the fire principle such as fevers, inflammatory diseases, and jaundice. Common symptoms seen in these types might include skin rashes, burning sensations, fevers, ulcerations, inflammation, or irritations such as colitis, conjunctivitis, or sore throats which can come and go.

The characteristics of pitta are hot, oily, light, mobile, dispersing, and liquid; any excess of any of these qualities can aggravate pitta. Summer is a time of heat and is the pitta season. Sunburn, poison ivy, prickly-type heat, and quick tempers are commonplace. These kinds of pitta disorders tend to calm down as the weather gets cooler, however. The dietary and lifestyle considerations place their emphasis on the need for coolness. Foods which are cooler, staying away from chili and spices, and cooler climates bode well for this type. People with excessive pitta need to exercise during the coolest time of the day.

Understanding Dietary Considerations

Here, the general food guidelines for balancing pitta include avoiding sour, salty, and overly pungent foods. Vegetarianism is suited to pitta types, and they should stay away from consuming alcohol, meat, eggs, and salty foods. To help calm their natural aggressiveness and compulsion, it's definitely beneficial to incorporate sweeter, cooler, and bitter foods and tastes into their diet plans.

Additionally, barley, rice, oats, and wheat are good grains for pitta dominant individuals, and vegetables should also aide a substantial part of their diet. Tomatoes, garlic, radishes, chilis, and raw onions should all be avoided. In fact, any vegetable that is too sour or hot will aggressively overload pitta, but most other vegetables will help to calm this dosha. Daikon radishes can be exceptionally cleansing for the liver when pitta is in balance but should be avoided at all other times. Salads and raw vegetables are good for pitta types in the spring and summer, as are the sweeter fruits. Sour fruits should be avoided, except limes, which can be utilized sparingly.

Animal foods, including eggs and seafood, should only be taken in moderation by pitta types. Protein foods such as chicken, turkey, rabbit, and venison are excellent. All legumes (apart from the red and yellow lentils) are wonderful in small amounts, with chickpeas and mung beans being superior here.

Most nuts and seeds have too much oil and are too hot for pitta. However, coconut is cooler, and sunflower seeds and pumpkin seeds are alright if only added in occasionally.

Smaller amounts of coconut, olive, and sunflower oils are also good for pitta. Sweet dairy products are beneficial for pitta, and include milk, unsalted butter, ghee, and softer, unsalted cheeses. Yogurt can be blended with spices with something sweet and water. And pitta types can use a sweetener more easily than the other 2 doshas because it relieves pitta. It's key that they avoid the hotter spices, but they can use cardamom, cinnamon, fennel, coriander, and turmeric broadly, with only small amounts of cumin and black pepper being utilized.

The use of coffee, alcohol, and tobacco products should be completely avoided. Black tea may also be used occasionally, with a touch of milk and a sprinkle of cardamom, as an example.

To Balance Pitta:

- Individual should avoid excessive heat
- Individual should avoid excessive oil
- Individual should avoid excessive steam
- Limit salt intake to a bare minimum
- Eat cooler, less spicy foods
- Exercise during the coolest time of the day

Describing Kapha

Kapha types are given much endurance ability, strength, and overall stamina. In balance, they tend to have sweet, kind, and loving characteristics, and be stable and grounded overall. Their skin is oily, but smooth. The kapha type may gain weight easily and have a slower metabolism than the other types. They tend to avoid exercise. They have thicker-type skin and their bodies and muscles are well developed. Their eyes are large and exceptionally attractive, with thicker, longer lashes and eyebrows. Kapha types have bowel movements more slowly than the other doshas, and their feces is usually softer, paler, and oilier. Their sweat is moderate, and sleep is usually deeper and more prolonged. Kapha types are attracted to sweeter, oilier; saltier foods, but their constitutions are most balanced by bitter, sour, and pungent food tastes.

In general, kapha people tend to be calmer, more tolerant, kind, and forgiving. However, they can become lethargic. While they may be slow to comprehend, their long-term memory is excellent. When out of order or off balance, kapha types may experience the archetypes of greed, envy, attachment, co-dependency, and possessiveness. All in all, kapha has a tendency toward groundedness, general stability, and attachment to ensure they can earn and hold onto money.

They are more likely to have diseases connected to the water principle, however. These include influenza, sinus issues, and other diseases involving mucous or the airways. They may battle with the feeling of sluggishness, have issues with excess weight gain, be prone to diabetes, have water retention, and/or headaches which can be commonplace. Kapha types can become more agitated as the moon gets fuller because there's a tendency for water retention to occur at this time. Winter is the best time for kapha and adhering to the kapha-balancing dietary and lifestyle changes are most important during the wintertime.

Understanding Dietary Considerations
Dietary guidelines for kapha people stress the need for bitter, sour, and pungent tastes. They direly need foods that will invigorate their minds while limiting their overall consumption of food. They should avoid dairy products and

fats of any type, especially fried or greasy foods, like those from takeaway stores.

The kapha dominant types need less grain than the pitta or vata types. As long as they haven't got an allergy, buckwheat and millet are the prime grains for them, followed by barley, corn, and rice too. Roasted or dry cooked grains are best suited here. Additionally, all types of vegetables are great for kapha, but leafy greens and vegetables grown above the ground (more often than root vegetables) are best. They do best when avoiding overly sweet, sour, or the juicier-type vegetables. Interestingly, kapha people can eat raw vegetables without much issue, although steamed or stir-fried are easier for them to digest. The overly sweet and sour-type fruits should be avoided. Dried fruits are preferable such as apricots, apples, cranberries, peaches, mangoes, and pears.

The kapha types rarely need animal foods, and dry-cooked, baked, roasted, and broiled are key when they do, but never fried versions of these. They can also eat eggs, chicken, rabbit, seafood, and venison. Kapha-dominant bodies don't need large amounts of protein, and overeating legumes is not advised, although these are better than meat because of the lack of fat. Black beans, mung beans, red lentils, and pinto beans are best for kapha types.

The heavier qualities within nuts and seeds can disturb and aggravate kapha types, including the oil found within them. Occasional sunflower and pumpkin seeds may be utilized, however. Corn, almond, safflower, or sunflower oils can be used in small amounts, and the same goes for dairy products. Here, kapha types should avoid the heavier, cooling, sweeter qualities of dairy. A little ghee for cooking and a small consumption of goat's milk is recommended.

Kapha types should definitely avoid sweets; the only sweetener they should use is raw honey, which is heating in its efficacy. Additionally, they can use all types of spices, except salt, with ginger and garlic being best for them. An individual with the dominant dosha of kapha, who has very little influence from the other 2 doshas, can benefit from the occasional use of stimulants such as coffee and tea. They are also not as harmed by tobacco or alcohol, however, but the use of stimulants is never recommended. If alcohol is enjoyed, wine is their best choice in moderation.

To Balance Kapha:

- Individuals should get plenty of exercise
- Individuals should avoid heavy foods
- Individuals should keep active
- Individuals should avoid dairy
- Individuals should avoid iced food and drinks
- Individuals should vary their routines
- Always avoid fatty and oily foods
- Eat lighter, drier foods
- Avoid daytime napping

Chapter 2: Understanding the Most Common Healing Methodologies

Ayurveda uses a range of treatments, including Panchakarma, as well as yoga, massage, acupuncture, and herbal medicine to encourage the individual's health and wellbeing.

The Panchakarma Definition

"Panchakarma" is a Sanskrit word which denotes 5 therapies or treatments used to rid the body of toxins, including the toxicity which may be there as a 'residue' left over from illness and/or disease. This prepares the body for its ability to accept the maximum benefits of nutrition, food, and exercise. There may be elaborate methods of 'purification' given by an Ayurvedic practitioner to alleviate the physical body from stress and toxins before a plan is set in place, however.

Panchakarma is therefore a specialized treatment consisting of 5 therapies which are meant to detoxify the body and balance the doshas.

Ayurveda may be able to treat a range of disorders including:

- Anxiety
- Depression
- Asthma
- Arthritis

- Digestive problems
- Eczema
- High blood pressure
- High cholesterol levels
- Rheumatoid arthritis
- Stress related disorders

Special considerations are herbs and rasa shastra medicines. As well as dietary considerations, herbal medicine is central to Ayurveda treatment.

Some safety issues to consider, include:

- Herbal medicines can be as potent as pharmaceutical drugs and it's true that inappropriate usage or overdose can occur

- Most complementary medicines have not been tested on pregnant women, breastfeeding mothers, or children

- Complementary medicines (such as herbs) can be bought without prescription, but there may be interactions with other medicines, either pharmaceutical or herbal in nature

- Products from other countries that are sold over the internet or brought from overseas may not be subject to the same laws or regulations as those sold in your current locality

- American research (in 2008) found that about 20% of Ayurvedic products bought online contained dangerous ingredients like lead, mercury, and arsenic in high enough quantities to be deemed toxic

- Rasa shastra medicines are found to be more likely than herb-only medicines to contain metals or have higher concentrations of metal
- Before buying or taking any complementary medicine, check the label for a (registered) code
- Avoid purchasing or using complementary medicines not registered, including those obtained from overseas
- If you are given a preparation by a friend or relative and you cannot identify the locality origin or ingredients, it's safer not to take the preparation
- Tell your practitioner about the Ayurvedic treatments you are having, as this will help to reduce the risk of adverse reactions
- Never stop taking your conventional medicine or alter the dose without the knowledge and approval of your practitioner

According to Ayurveda, an individual's health is not defined as being completely disease-free. It's the state of normalcy of the 3 doshas of vata, pitta, and kapha which broadly allow for the balance of the nervous, the metabolic, and the nutritive system.

These 3 key doshas keep the physical body, the mind, and the emotions in balance. A disease is manifested when the balance or disorder between the doshas is disturbed or disordered.

Having an Ayurvedic cleanse draws out the toxins from the body, also pulling out excess vata, pitta, and kapha from the tissues into the digestive tract and in order to eliminate them more fully and easily. This, in turn, unblocks the imbalance and restores overall balance. This cleanse is known as Panchakarma and is a method of cleansing the body of all unwanted waste after lubricating the body first. This treatment is highly beneficial as it includes preventive and curative actions for various illnesses, sicknesses, and/or diseases.

The Key Benefits of Panchakarma

- Clearing toxins from the entire system
- Balancing the doshas
- Healing the digestive system
- Enhancing the immunity
- Decreasing stress
- Anti-aging benefits
- Improved skin shine
- Weight loss, if necessary
- Deep, peaceful relaxation
- A meditative outlook on the individual's life
- Enhanced mindfulness

The Panchakarma Treatment Procedure

The process of Panchakarma involves following 3 steps:

1. Poorva Karma

This procedure is required before the main treatment and is used to soften the tissues so that the lipid-soluble toxins deposited into them are liquefied and can flow back to the digestive tract. From there, they may be eliminated. This treatment prepares the individual both mentally and physically for the main procedure of Panchakarma.

Pachan Karma

This improves digestion with herbs and fasting so that the individual can digest the clarified butter (ghee) which is provided to liquefy the fat-soluble toxins.

Snehan Karma

The prepared medicated ghee is given to the individual in increasing doses, and this is done in order to aggravate and liquefy the fat-soluble toxins. These toxins are deposited within the deeper tissues.

Swedan Karma

Now a full body steam bath is given to the individual so that there can be an opening up of the bodily channels. Here, the heat will liquefy the toxins further. This facilitates their movement from the tissues and into the digestive tract.

2. Pradhan Karma

This is the 5-step procedure which is highly unique, depending on the needs of the individual, age, digestive strength, current immune system, and some other poignant factors. This exceptionally intense Panchakarma procedure can only be done under the guidance of an Ayurvedic practitioner.

The 5 karmas to cleanse the complete body:

Vamanam: The Therapeutic Emesis

This is induced vomiting which helps clear the upper GI tract to the duodenum (end of the stomach), and also a part of the respiratory tract.

Virechanam: The Purgation

The induced purgation clears the GI tract from the duodenum to the exit.

Anuvasana: The Enema with Medicated Oil

Here, the oil enema helps to lubricate the rectal area and to cleanse the lipid soluble waste out through the anus.

Nasyam: The Nasal Inhalation

This is the nasal inhalation using medicated substances which will help to clear the respiratory tract and the para nasal sinus areas.

3. Paschaat Karma: The After-Therapy Dietary Regime

This is an after-therapy dietary regime to restore the body's digestive and absorptive capacity to its normalcy. It includes rejuvenation treatments, lifestyle management, dietary management, and an intake of herbal supplements.

Sansarjan Karma: The Food Therapy After Detoxification

This is food therapy after the detoxification occurs, which helps to gradually increase the individual's diet from liquids to semi-solids, and then to a normal diet.

Rasayan Adi Prayogam: The Rejuvenation Therapy

This is a rejuvenating Rasayan therapy which aids in boosting natural immunity and enhancing the individual's general wellbeing.

Shaman Chikitsa: The Pacification Therapy

This is a pacification therapy with herbs and lifestyle management combined.

Overall, a Panchakarma procedure is designed uniquely for an individual after a thorough physical examination and a pulse diagnosis. So, there's really no universal system as such. These mentioned treatments can take a minimum of 1 week and may last as long as 3 weeks.

Almost anyone can benefit from a Panchakarma procedure, and this is because the body is constantly creating toxins on a regular basis. These are the signs to know if you need a detox:

- A thickly layered coating on the tongue
- Feeling tired throughout the day, especially after mealtimes
- Body aches and/or pains
- Uncontrollable cravings for foods
- A foggy mind or lack of clarity
- Bad breath, intense body odor, and/or flatulence
- Constipation or diarrhea

The purpose of Panchakarma is purification or Sodhana. If a disease is treated with the Sodhana approach it doesn't come back. Therefore, the Panchakarma Sodhana is the ultimate way to heal and rebalance the physical body.

Certain Panchakarma procedures are not suitable for some health problems, however, and some procedures should not be performed on children, pregnant women, or the elderly or aged. Additionally, Panchakarma treatments should only ever be performed by qualified and experienced Ayurvedic practitioners.

Known Side Effects of Panchakarma

Common side effects of Panchakarma include general fatigue, a feeling of malaise, headaches, congestion, and general illness symptoms. An initial increase in the symptoms may also occur as a side effect, at first.

It's also noteworthy that as Panchakarma seeks to release stored emotional problems, some patients can experience mental disturbances and depression during the course of the prescribed treatment.

A More in Depth Look at Dietary Changes & Herbal Remedies

Herbal medicine, including the combination of herbs with metals, minerals, or gems (or rasha shastra medicines) that can take the form of pellets, tablets and/or powders of various colors and scents.

Consistency with regards to composition and biological activity are essential requirements for the safe and effective use of any type of therapeutic agents. Quality is truly the critical ingredient for safety and efficacy of botanical-type medicines, but sometimes preparations rarely meet the standards necessary. And this relates to procedures and markers for assessing and testing their strength. This relates to the strength of botanical raw materials or extracts from formulations of multiple substances combined.

Similarly, like China, efforts are needed to raise the image of Ayurvedic medicines in the global business model. The government of India has inserted GMP regulations for traditional systems of medicines to improve the quality and standard of Ayurvedic drugs in pharmacies. Other new rules regarding essential infrastructure, manpower, and control with regards to quality requirements came into force from the year 2000 and make up part of the *Drugs and Cosmetics Act* of 1940. Interestingly too, the licensing of Ayurvedic medicine is also governed under the same act. Additionally, *Ayurvedic Patent and Proprietary* medicines need to be made up of only the ingredients mentioned in the recommended books as is specified within the Act.

Standardization of Herbal Medicines

Standardization of herbal drugs is not just a logically solved operation for identification, it actually comprises of total information and controls which mostly guarantee the consistent composition of all herbals. A viable example of this is a polyherbal formulation by Artrex® which was made for the treatment of arthritis and contains 4 botanicals. The formulation is standardized using modern scientific tools, including known markers, and has been granted a U.S. patent.

The Indian herbal drug industry needs to ensure measures of standardized, authentic raw components, and those which are free from toxic contaminants. Improving technologies which are processed, adhering to GMP compliance, and maintaining in-process quality control for manufacturing quality herbal products is key. There's also the need for evidence of an herbal formula's therapeutic efficacy, safety adherents, and its overall shelf life. Such approaches remain key to the global promotion of Ayurveda.

Government Policies

In both China and India, formal training is an ongoing part of the national health program, which helps in maintaining quality standards in health care delivery and efficacy. Science-based approaches were utilized in China and about 95% of general hospitals in the country have traditional medicine departments, which is something new to Western culture.

The government of India also has expressed support and encouragement for the rolling out of alternative medicines. A separate department for *Indian Systems of Medicine and Homeopathy* (ISM&H) is also known as AYUSH (Ayurveda, Yoga, Unani, Siddha, Homoeopathy). Its priorities include valuable education, standardization, enhancement and availability of raw materials, ongoing research and development, added information, communication, and a bigger involvement in the national system for delivering health care. *The Central Council for Indian Medicine* oversees training institutes and teaching, while *Central Council for Research* in Ayurveda and Siddha allows and promotes with interdisciplinary research.

Some products are being added into family welfare programs of the government under the *World Bank* project. These medicinal drugs are directed at common diseases like anemia, and some pregnancy complaints like edema during pregnancy, including pregnancy postpartum problems such as pain, and uterine and abdominal complications. Other help is quantified for difficulties with lactation, nutritional deficiencies, and childhood diarrhea.

The government has established 10 testing laboratories and is upgrading pre-existing laboratories to provide high quality evidence through documentation, and to licensing authorities for the safety and quality of these herbal medicines. This replaces the earlier system of testing that was considered as being mostly unreliable. In the year 2002, the *Council for Scientific and Industrial Research* launched a research program under the scheme with *New Millennium Indian Technology Leadership Initiative* in Ayurveda, identifying 3 disease areas including arthritis, diabetes, and hepatic disorders, which affect large numbers of the Indian population annually.

Much of Indian botanical sources and their medicinal properties (like turmeric) have been patented. This has been done in many cases by way of claiming innovations that were already popular within the public domain. Necessary measures to protect intellectual property are important, however, and this is due to the retrieval and contesting of patents being a very costly and time-consuming affair. And so, the government of India established the *Traditional Knowledge Digital Library* for traditional medicinal plants, which will also lead to a *Traditional Knowledge Resource Classification* in the future. Joining this to the internationally accepted *International Patent Classification* system will mean bridging the gap between the knowledge contained in an old Sanskrit text, and a patent examiner. It might integrate broadly scattered and distributed references in retrievable form, so it will be a major asset to modern research in the developing world.

Research is Mesmerizing for the Future of Ayurveda

Natural products' extracts of therapeutic direction are of major importance as key ingredients of structural and chemical diversity. A recent review on national pharmacopoeias from several countries reveals at least 110 distinct chemical substances from different plants that have the capacity as lifesaving drugs. This has been ascertained through chemical and pharmacological screening of only 6-7% of the total plant species. Its beginning stages are quite eye-opening, in fact.

Untapped, hidden wealth in the flora needs to be found and studied to cure diseases like AIDS, cancer, neurological disorders, diabetes, etc. Recently, the NIH began extensive research for anti-inflammatory compounds from turmeric, ginger, and Boswellia. This occurred because of the foundational study of Ayurvedic knowledge. Screening of different plants for anticancer components is also in progress with references of experiential data from traditional systems. The world is an 'oyster' of drugs is definitely the theme where Ayurveda is concerned.

India has world-class expertise and facilities for organic synthetics, as well as isolation and structure building. It can also handle biological screening, toxicological testing, and the area of pharmacokinetics. This is supplemented by the knowledge for the continued development of agrotechnology, and for the ability towards the cultivation of medicinal plants.

It's also true, that industry participation to ensure successful upscaling and implementation of technology is building. There's a generation of leads with structural diversities through the propelled creation of natural product libraries, and via the identification of proper targets, including proper validation and optimization.

India has extensive research institutes like the *Central Drug Research Institute* (CDRI), *Central Institute of Medicinal and Aromatic Plants,* and the *National Botanical Research Institute.* Additionally, *Regional Research Laboratories* (RRL), in Jammu, Bhubaneshwar and Jorhat, with a *National Chemical Laboratory* at Pune, which routinely researches various types of medicinal plants.

Supporting Systems

Apart from the drug manufacturing companies, many other supporting industries also play important roles in the well-needed commerce of traditional medicine. There's a whole array of industries which are the collectors and breeders, the dealers of the plant materials, the processors, and the manufacturing industry too. Then there are the practitioners of traditional medicine and the consumers who buy it all.

Currently, Indian systems of medicine use more than 1000 medicinal plants, and most are collected from the wilderness. More than 50 species are in great demand right now. The wilderness of India is rich in these plants and the tribes who live there mainly depend on this trade for their own livelihood. Here, the adequate availability of quality and raw materials free from adulterants at reasonable prices has become a huge problem for the industry, and the demand for the raw materials is increasing annually.

Unfortunately, very few efforts have been made by either the government or by industry to seriously study the supply and demand modelling. Like China, India needs to follow GAPs to ensure the use of correct raw materials and include the entire life cycle including the needs allowable for harvesting, processing, transportation, and for long-term storage. Comparatively, the Chinese government has built more than 100 research facilities and encouraged private companies to build over 600 planting bases for herbs which are in great demand. India might do well to look at the China model for future sustainability as well as the supply, demand, and infrastructure needs related to this branch of industry.

Drug Therapy

Many drugs have entered the international market via the exploration of ethnopharmacology as well as traditional medicine. Progress in genomics and proteomics has brought about new gateways in therapeutics and drug discovery, as well as its development. Ayurvedic medicine can benefit from this, just like other traditional medicines have.

A better understanding of the human genome has helped in allowing for the scientific basis of individual variation. Drug targets have grown during the last decade, but the industry remains target-rich, overall.

TIM (Traditional Indian Medicine) and TCM (Traditional Chinese Medicine) have many generations' observations that have well-organized and documented data. And although various scientific studies have been done on a variety of Indian-inspired botanicals, a considerably smaller number of marketable drugs have entered the evidence-based therapeutics.

In comparison, China has successfully promoted its own therapies and drugs very well. Some of these include ginseng, ma huang, and gingko, with scientific evidence accepted on a global scale. Approaching integrative medicine by selective incorporation of the elements of TCM as well as the modern methods of diagnosis has achieved a great success in China. Another great potential model which might work well for India and Ayurveda medicine on the global scale.

India, however, must ensure a clearer policy for such integration without compromise on the strategies that are truly science-based. Efforts are needed to establish and validate research evidence regarding both the safety and practice of Ayurvedic medicines.

Pharmacoeconomic studies on TIM and TCM are rare but can help in understanding cost efficacy and the cost benefits of traditional medicine. In all attempts, TCM examples would aide India at various levels, including making policies, utilizing quality standards, including integration practices, using viable research models, and the complementary allowance where public health is kept as the central focus. Both TIM and TCM are great traditions with a bold philosophical basis, and could play an integral role in newer therapies, including further drug discovery, and developmental processes overall.

Worldwide Changes in Favor of Natural Drug Therapies

Ayurveda is the traditional Indian medicine (TIM), and traditional Chinese medicine (TCM) both remain the most ancient living traditions. These are 2 practices with sound experiential, philosophical, and experimental bases. In Western medicine, the increased side effects, the lack of curative treatment for several chronic diseases, the high cost of new drugs, continued microbial resistance, and emerging diseases are some reasons for the increased public interest in complementary and alternative medicines. Ayurveda is one of them.

Many pharmaceutical companies have changed their strategies to be in favor of natural product drug development and discovery. For instance, in Europe, there has been a renewed inclusion of drug discovery based on natural product chemistry. In the Asia-Pacific region, some pharmaceutical companies have comprehensive structures and the innate capabilities necessary for natural product-based drug discovery.

China has successfully promoted its own therapies internationally, albeit with a science-based approach. Growing popularity of TCM can be seen by the rapid increase in the number of licensed Chinese medicine providers within the United States. The Chinese government has pledged to build several exports which are oriented by the TCM giants in the coming decades.

Continuous efforts in promotion of the indigenous therapies by China have put TCM in a wonderful position. Global acceptance of Ayurveda is on the increase as well, and there's also been a steady rise in the demand for medicinal plants from India, too.

The Western scientific community views traditional medicines cautiously, and always points out the concerns related to research, development, efficacy, and quality.

Interestingly though, the global pharmaceutical market was worth a whopping $550 billion U.S. in 2004 and is rising continually over time. The herbal industry shares about $62 billion U.S. with good growth potential. The *World Bank* reports trade in medicinal-type plants, raw materials, and is growing at an annual growth rate of close to 20%.

Within the European community, botanical medicine represents an important inclusivity of the pharmaceutical market, where the sector is also growing rapidly worldwide. In 2001, $17.8 billion was used in the United States on dietary supplements, and $4.2 billion of it was for botanical remedies alone.

In India, the value of botanicals is about $10 billion U.S. per year, with the annual export of approximately $1.1 billion. Meanwhile, China's annual herbal drug production is worth approximately $48 billion with an export of $3.6 billion.

At present, the United States is the largest market for Indian botanical products, making up for around 55% of the total exports. After this, Japan, Hong Kong, Korea, and Singapore are the major importers of TCM, taking over a 60% share of China's botanical drugs export.

Worldwide, there have been major efforts to monitor quality and regulate the growing industry of herbal drugs and traditional medicines. Health authorities and governments of various nations have taken an active approach in providing standardized medications which have botanical properties, too. Interestingly, the United States Congress accelerated rapid growth in the nutraceutical market with the addition of the *Dietary Supplement Health and Education Act* in 1994. Additionally, the *US Food and Drug Administration* (FDA) published the *International Conference on Harmonization* guidance *Common Technical Document,* and this served to address concerns related to quality of medicines that also includes herbals, too.

The National Center for Complementary and Alternative Medicine has the mission to explore complementary and alternative healing practices in the context of true science, to maintain its support of sophisticated research, to train researchers, and also give information to the public on the modalities that do work, and explain the scientific rationale of all underlying discoveries.

The U.S. center is committed to exploring and funding all types of therapies for which there is sufficient data, a compelling public health need, and by including ethical justifications. The global scenario shows both promise and challenges presented by the traditional medicines.

It's clear that India needs to identify the extent to which Ayurvedic therapeutics is safe, including showing this scientifically for global acceptance. Using trusted research facilities and trusted science-based approaches will be key to extend the global market as a practice, and as a trusted branch of ancient (but modernized) medicine. This will also appeal to millions who are seeking alternative therapies and treatment options within the current modern world.

Basic Principles of TIM and TCM

Ayurveda and TCM have many similarities. The focus of both the systems is on the individual, rather than on disease. Both systems aim to promote overall health and enhance the quality of the individual's life, with therapeutic strategies for the treatment of specific diseases or symptoms.

Almost half of the botanical sources used as medicines have similarities when looking at TIM and TCM comparatively, and both systems have similar philosophies geared towards enabling the classification of individuals through characteristics, materials, and diseases.

TCM considers the human as being at the center of the cosmos, as an 'antenna' between the celestial and earthly elements. The elements of water, earth, metal, wood, and fire are the 5 elements of the material world. The world is a single unit, and its flow gives rise to yin and yang, the two main aspects.

The actual meaning of the term yin and yang is 'opposites,' being the positive and the negative polarities. The Chinese believe that yin and yang is not absolute, but relative. This is similar with the modern view of homeostasis, where yin and yang are interchanged to meet the view that yang declines and yin rises, or yang is raised up to produce a decline of yin.

The 4 bodily humors (qi, blood, moisture, and essence) and the internal organ systems (known as zang fu) play an exceptional role in balancing the yin and yang within the physical body. True formation, maintenance, and circulation of these energies are essential for health and wellbeing, in fact. When the 2 energies fall out of harmony, this is when disease develops. The practitioner takes into account this concept while treating the individual. Drugs or herbs are used to correct this imbalance of yin-yang within the human physical body in TCM.

Ayurveda believes that the universe is made up of combinations of the 5 elements (pancha mahabhutas). These are known as being akasha (ether), vayu (air), teja (fire), aap (water), and prithvi (earth).

These 5 elements can be seen to exist in the physical universe at all areas of life, and in both organic and inorganic things. In biological systems, such as human beings, elements are coded into 3 forces, and these govern all life processes.

The 3 forces (kapha, pitta and vata) are the 3 doshas or simply the tridosha. Each of the doshas is composed of one or two elements as we discovered earlier. The tridosha regulates every physiological and psychological process within the living organism. The interplay among them determines the qualities and conditions of the individual.

A balanced state of the 3 doshas creates balance and health, whereas an imbalance, which might be an excess (known as vriddhi) or a deficiency (known as kshaya), manifests as a sign or a symptom of disease.

Both TCM and TCI have their pros and cons, just as any type of medicine does. It's important to understand that Ayurvedic medicine is done by a practitioner, a professional who has studied and is competent within the field.

Below is a list of things to remember, especially where the ingestion of medicines is concerned. And as with any practice, you need to look at the pros and cons before deciding upon a therapy which is right for you.

This book is made as an introduction to Ayurvedic medicine and reflects the pros and cons, including some comparisons, so that you can make an informed choice about your own health, overall. It's vital to have enough knowledge so that you can make an informed decision for you or your loved ones.

The ancient practice of Ayurveda has been around for many thousands of years, and so it might be of interest to you to compare it with other practices, including Western medicine and TCM. In this way, you'll have enough knowledge to make an informed decision on what you might like to choose.

Remember to look at the *References* and the *Suggested Reading* list at the end of this title. Some of the knowledge given there is highly valuable.

Important Things to Remember

- Ayurveda or Ayurvedic medicine is a system of traditional medicine which is native to India

43

- Treatment options are varied and are best spoken about with a professional Ayurvedic practitioner
- There have been cases of lead poisoning as a result of taking Ayurvedic treatments imported from India, so always buy from a registered, trusted retailer
- Always check with your own practitioner before starting complementary therapies or medicines, and never stop taking your conventional medicine or alter the dosage without the knowledge and approval of your current practitioner
- Some herbal medicines can interact with other herbal medicines and prescribed pharmaceutical drugs

Chapter 3: The Incorporation of Dietary Considerations Using Ayurveda

"You Are What You Eat!" in Ayurvedic Medicine

We've all heard of that really famous saying, "You are what you eat!" The basics of Ayurvedic nutrition is that *we* are the result of not only *what* we eat, but *how* and *why,* and even *when* we eat.

Ayurveda is a balanced approach to eating that suggests we eat thoughtfully, healthfully, and that we do this with expressed gratitude. Our diets should always be super fresh, easily digestible, prepared with care, and alluring to all of our senses. All in all, we should eat a variety of foods, herbs, and spices that are visually appealing, aromatic, and flavorful.

As we already know, Ayurveda recognizes 6 exponential tastes, and believes we should have all these tastes within our diets every day. The 6 tastes have qualities that will either increase or decrease the doshas.

Sweet is heavier, sour is moister, salty is warmer, bitter is colder, pungent is hotter, and astringent is dryer. In fact, foods with qualities like the dosha qualities will increase it, and foods with the opposite qualities to the dosha will decrease it. The need for balance is key. Ayurveda also accentuates eating these tastes in a particular order, from the sweetest to the most astringent, which means we can eat dessert first to feel satisfied, and to digest our food correctly. The most interesting thing is, by not having all 6 tastes it can lead to big cravings, a thorough lack of energy, small or large weight gain, illness, and/or disease.

Ayurveda encourages individuals to eat seasonally, organically, mindfully, and healthfully. The way we eat and relate to food can be linked to other aspects of our lives. If our food is filled with life force (known as prana), then we'll have the health and energy necessary to live our lives to the fullest, and do it healthfully, too.

A Revision of the Doshas with Relation to Food

At first, let's take a moment to go back to some of the key elements we looked at for each dosha. It's important to highlight what we already know.

Highlighting the Dietary Considerations for Vata

For vata, the individual should include warm and well-cooked foods. An individual should have smaller meals 3 or 4 times a day, and can snack as needed, while still maintaining a 2-hour gap between each smaller meal. Regularity for mealtimes is important for the dominant vata type. Great ideas can be soups, stews, and casseroles too. They can use more oil in cooking their foods than the other 2 dosha types and enjoy far better digestion if they limit their intake of raw foods.

While cooked vegetables are best for vata, the occasional salad with a good oily or creamy dressing is great. Foods such as tomatoes, potatoes, peppers, spinach, and eggplants should be avoided if the vata dominant has aching or stiff joints or

46

muscles. Sweet, ripe, and juicy-type fruits are excellent for the dominant vata types. Additionally, dried fruits like raw apples and cranberries should be avoided. Fruit should always be eaten by itself and on an empty stomach.

Many vata types can satisfy their need for protein by the consistent use of dairy products, and they may also utilize eggs, chicken, fresh fish, turkey, and venison too. Legumes are difficult for this type to digest properly and should be consumed in minimal quantities by those trying to balance out vata. Additionally, legumes should be the split type and soaked very well before cooking. Cooking them with minimal oil and spices, like garlic, turmeric, cumin, coriander, and ginger will help prevent vata from becoming off balance or disordered.

It's also important to note that nuts and seeds are especially good for vata but are best used as butters or in milks. All dairy products are good for vata with harder cheeses needing to be eaten sparingly.

Additionally, spices are great, but should not be overused. Vatas can have about a half a glass of wine, diluted with water, either during or after a meal. Since vata people are prone to addiction, they should always avoid processed sugar, caffeine, and tobacco products. Eat warmer foods and spices.

Highlighting the Dietary Considerations for Pitta

For pitta, the general food guidelines for balancing pitta include avoiding sour, salty, and overly pungent foods. Vegetarianism is suited to pitta types, and they should stay away from consuming alcohol, meat, eggs, and salty foods. To help calm their natural aggressiveness and compulsion, it's definitely beneficial to incorporate sweeter, cooler, and bitter foods and tastes into their diet plans.

Additionally, barley, rice, oats, and wheat are good grains for pitta dominant individuals, and vegetables should also aide a substantial part of their diet. Tomatoes, garlic, radishes, chilis, and raw onions should all be avoided. In fact, any vegetable that is too sour or hot will aggressively overload pitta, but most other vegetables will help to calm this dosha. Daikon radishes can be exceptionally cleansing for the liver when pitta is in balance but should be avoided at all other times. Salads and raw vegetables are good for pitta types in the spring and summer, as are the sweeter fruits. Sour fruits should be avoided, except limes, which can be utilized sparingly.

Animal foods, including eggs and seafood, should only be taken in moderation by pitta types. Protein foods such as chicken, turkey, rabbit, and venison are excellent. All legumes (apart from the red and yellow lentils) are wonderful in small amounts, with chickpeas and mung beans being superior here.

Most nuts and seeds have too much oil and are too hot for pitta. However, coconut is cooler, and sunflower seeds and pumpkin seeds are alright if only added in occasionally. Smaller amounts of coconut, olive, and sunflower oils are also good for pitta. Sweet dairy products are beneficial for pitta, and include milk, unsalted butter, ghee, and softer, unsalted cheeses. Yogurt can be blended with spices with something sweet and water. And pitta types can use a sweetener more easily than the other 2 doshas because it relieves pitta. It's key that they avoid the hotter spices, but they can use cardamom, cinnamon, fennel, coriander, and turmeric broadly, with only small amounts of cumin and black pepper being utilized.

The use of coffee, alcohol, and tobacco products should be completely avoided. Black tea may also be used occasionally, with a touch of milk and a sprinkle of cardamom, as an example. The individual should avoid excessive heat with regards to foods and temperature. The individual should avoid excessive oil. The individual should limit salt intake to a bare minimum, and eat cooler, less spicy foods.

Highlighting the Dietary Considerations for Kapha

For kapha, there's the need to include bitter, sour, and pungent tastes. They direly need foods that will invigorate their minds while limiting their overall consumption of food. They should avoid dairy products and fats of any type, especially fried or greasy foods, like those from takeaway stores.

The kapha dominant types need less grain than the pitta or vata types. As long as they haven't got an allergy, buckwheat and millet are the prime grains for them, followed by barley, corn, and rice too. Roasted or dry cooked grains are best suited here. Additionally, all types of vegetables are great for kapha, but leafy greens and vegetables grown above the ground (more often than root vegetables) are best. They do best when avoiding overly sweet, sour, or the juicier-type vegetables. Interestingly, kapha people can eat raw vegetables without much issue, although steamed or stir-fried are easier for them to digest. The overly sweet and sour-type fruits should be avoided. Dried fruits are preferable such as apricots, apples, cranberries, peaches, mangoes, and pears.

The kapha types rarely need animal foods, and dry-cooked, baked, roasted, and broiled are key when they do, but never fried versions of these. They can also eat eggs, chicken, rabbit, seafood, and venison. Kapha-dominant bodies don't need large amounts of protein, and overeating legumes is not advised, although these are better than meat because of the lack of fat. Black beans, mung beans, red lentils, and pinto beans are best for kapha types.

The heaver qualities within nuts and seeds can disturb and aggravate kapha types, including the oil found within them. Occasional sunflower and pumpkin seeds may be utilized, however. Corn, almond, safflower, or sunflower oils can be used in small amounts, and the same goes for dairy products. Here, kapha types should avoid the heavier, cooling, sweeter qualities of dairy. A little ghee for cooking and a small consumption of goat's milk is recommended.

Kapha types should definitely avoid sweets; the only sweetener they should use is raw honey, which is heating in its efficacy. Additionally, they can use all types of spices, except salt, with ginger and garlic being best for them. An individual with the dominant dosha of kapha, who has very little influence from the other 2 doshas, can benefit from the occasional use of stimulants such as coffee and tea. They are also not as harmed by tobacco or alcohol, however, but the use of stimulants is never recommended. If alcohol is enjoyed, wine is their best choice in moderation. Individuals should avoid heavy foods. Individuals should avoid iced food and drinks. Always avoid fatty and oily foods. Eat lighter, drier foods.

The Food Types

The types of food we're dealing with here are in categories. There are sweet, salty, bitter, sour, astringent, and spicy too. This is very similar to TCM (Traditional Chinese Medicine).

Sometimes, each food might look like it should be in an alternative category, however, it's the way the food is ingested and understood inside the body. So, if it seems as though an item of food should belong elsewhere, that's because its taste is perceived after being eaten. A great example of this is a lemon which is an acidic food, but when it hits the stomach it becomes alkaline.

Let's take a look at these categories in detail now:

Sour Foods

- Beef
- Yoghurt
- Barbecue sauce
- Turkey
- Vinegar
- Tomatoes
- Sprouts
- Sausages
- Sour cream
- Salad dressing
- Salami
- Bread

- Chicken
- Freshwater fish
- Liver
- Raw fruit
- Fruit juices
- Mayonnaise
- Red meats
- Pickles

Bitter Foods

- Green vegetables
- Artichokes
- Asparagus
- Tea
- Turnips
- Bamboo shoots
- Bok choy
- Cocoa
- Coffee
- Gelatin
- Green vegetables
- Heart (any animal)
- Leeks
- Mushrooms
- Broccoli
- Cauliflower
- Celery
- Gelatin
- Avocados
- Bitter melon

Sweet Foods

- Oatmeal
- Milk
- Lettuce
- Beans
- Kale
- Ice cream
- Honey
- Eggplant
- Cucumber
- Corn
- Cream
- Dried fruit
- Coconut
- Carrots
- Candy
- Cakes
- Canned fruits
- Brazil nuts
- Almonds
- Beans
- Bran
- Wheat
- Walnuts
- Sweet potatoes
- Peanuts
- Peas
- Rice
- Squash
- Sugar
- Sunflower seeds

- Sweets
- Pecans
- Soda
- Starchy foods

Astringent Foods

- Leafy greens
- Green bananas
- Cranberries
- Salt
- High potassium foods
- Pomegranates
- Various Herbs

Spicy Foods

- Wine
- Basil
- Cayenne pepper
- Chili
- Garlic
- Curry
- Dill
- Ginger
- Lung (any animal)
- Garlic
- Mustard
- Mint
- Rhubarb
- Pepper
- Parsley

- Oregano
- Onions
- Mustard
- Time
- Truffles
- Aniseed

Salty Foods

- Bones
- Prepared beef
- Canned foods
- Cheese
- Egg
- Salt-water fish
- Butter
- Frozen foods
- Tofu
- Shellfish
- Seaweed
- Most processed foods
- Margarine
- Pickled olives
- Kidneys (any animal)
- Caviar

The Importance of Ayurveda

Ayurveda, which we know comes from the ancient Vedic texts, is a 5000-year-old medical philosophy and practice, and is based upon the idea that we're made up of different types of energy. The doshas in Ayurveda describe the dominant mind/body state. We know these to be: vata, pitta, and kapha.

While all 3 doshas are present in everyone, Ayurveda states that we each have a dominant dosha that's unwavering from the time we were conceived, and ideally an equal (although often fluctuating) balance between the other 3 doshas. When the doshas are balanced and ordered, the individual can be truly healthy, but when they are unbalanced or disordered, the individual may develop illness or disease, which is usually shown first as skin issues, poor digestion, the onset of insomnia, grumpiness or irritability, and anxiety, too.

In India and other parts of the East, including Nepal, Ayurveda is thought to be both important and significant medicine. With schooling that's equivalent with a Western medical degree, Ayurveda can be lifechanging, to say the least. Different to Western medicine, a basic understanding goes beyond just a physical exam. An Ayurvedic practitioner will take the individual's pulse, check the tongue, and assess the individual's overall appearance (among other things), and then ask a series of questions about how the individual handles and responds to various scenarios, too.

The principle that recognizes that each human being is born with unique combinations of doshas is also key, and that this natural order and state of balance is what's responsible for the innate physical, mental, and emotional differences among individuals. By identifying and maintaining an individual's dominant dosha, Ayurveda can help individuals to create their own state of ideal health. Let's take a look at each dosha again, with some more characteristics and additional information, so then we might get to know each one more intimately for the purposes of this chapter.

Vata: Air & Space

These individuals tend to be dreamier and can be anxious but have active minds. They speak quickly and are likely to have joints that crack. Vata influences the movement of thoughts, feelings, prana, nerve impulses, and fluids in the body.

Some words which identify this dosha include irregular, cold, light, dry, rough, moving, quick, and everchanging. Vata governs movement of the body, the activities of the nervous system, and the process of elimination (toileting). Vata also influences the other doshas. Vatas seem to always be on the go and have energetic and creative minds. When vatas are in order (balanced), they are lively and enthusiastic.

Their thin, light frame is pronounced, and they have excellent adaptability. Their energy seems to come in bursts, and they're likely to experience sudden bouts of fatigue after a time, however. These individuals typically have cold hands and feet; they sleep lightly, and their digestion can be overly sensitive. When they're disordered (imbalanced), these individuals may experience weight loss, arthritis, constipation, weakness, restlessness, and/or aches and pains.

Vata individuals generally love excitement and new or fun experiences. They're quick to get angry, but also to forgive. They're energetic, flexible, and ingenious. They also take the initiative and are great conversationalists. When disordered (imbalanced), they're prone to worry, becoming anxious, may suffer from nervousness, and often get insomnia. When they feel stressed or overwhelmed, their response is usually, "What did *I* do wrong?"

Vatas should follow the guidelines below:

1. Maintain a regular daily routine and keep exercise both gentle and regulated.

2. Find time for rest and to nurture the self. Be in a safe, calm, and comforting environment.

3. Have regular Ayurvedic massages which are grounding and soothing.

4. Avoid overly cold and windy conditions, as well as overly dry climates.

5. Minimize travel and too much movement. They should also avoid loud and noisy places with crowds and too much talking.

6. Keep warm and get adequate sleep each day.

Vata is known as the colder and dryer dosha, so warming and nourishing foods with a moderately heavy texture are great, plus added butter and fat are excellent for stability. They should choose the saltier, sour, and sweeter tastes, as well as soothing and satisfying foods. So, warm milk, cream, butter, soups, stews, hot cereals, freshly baked bread, raw nuts, and nut butters are excellent for vatas, if they have no allergies to any of these mentioned products. Additionally, hot, or herbal tea with snacks in the late afternoon are key. All sweet fruits (extra-ripe are best) are good for these individuals. Warm drinks or hot water are best too.

Cold foods like salads, iced drinks, raw vegetables, and greens are not recommended where vata is dominant. Avoiding drinks with too much caffeine, and candy too, as these will disorder (unbalance) this dosha. Avoiding unripe fruits is also paramount, and this is because they're too astringent for these individuals.

The Best Vegetables for Vata (cooked)

Asparagus, carrots, beets, cucumber, garlic, green beans, onions, sweet potatoes, radishes, and turnips.

The Vegetables to Have in Moderation for Vata (cooked)

Broccoli, cauliflower, cabbage, Brussel sprouts, peppers, tomatoes, celery, potatoes, eggplant, leafy green vegetables, mushrooms, peas, sprouts, and zucchini. Avoid all raw vegetables.

The Best Fruits (Well-Ripened) for Vata

Bananas, cherries, apricots, avocados, berries, coconut, fresh figs, grapefruit, lemons, grapes, mangoes, sweet melons, peaches, sour oranges, papaya, pineapple, plums, and stewed fruits.

The Fruits in Moderation for Vata

Cranberries, pomegranates, and pears. Avoid dried fruits in general, and all unripe fruit.

The Best Grains for Vata

Oats (cooked), and rice (cooked).

The Grains in Moderation for Vata

Wheat, dry oat, buckwheat, corn, barley, and millet.

The Best Dairy for Vata

All dairy products are acceptable.

The Best Meat for Vata

Chicken, turkey, and seafood, but all in smaller quantities.

The Meat in Moderation for Vata

Red meat.

The Best Beans for Vata

Chickpeas, pink lentils, tofu (small amounts), and mung beans.

The Beans in Moderation for Vata

Kidney beans and black beans.

The Best Oils for Vata

Sesame, olive, and ghee are excellent.

The Sweeteners for Vata

All sweeteners can be utilized.

The Nuts & Seeds for Vata

All nuts and seeds are acceptable in small amounts. Almonds are excellent, however.

The Herbs & Spices for Vata

Cardamom, cinnamon, cumin, ginger, cloves, and garlic are all good for these individuals.

Vata should avoid using spices in large quantities. Minimizing or avoiding all bitter and astringent herbs and spices such as coriander seed, parsley, fenugreek, and thyme. Saffron and turmeric should only be used in moderation.

Pitta: Fire & a Little Water

Pittas have more fire in them than the other dosha types. They have better appetites and better digestion, too. They can handle the cold better, and this is because they're hot-headed as a general characteristic. They're naturally aggressive and also impatient, but they're super intelligent and very sharp. Since these individuals have strong and efficient digestion, they can eat just about everything. Most of these individuals get into trouble by the continued use of too much salt, however, including the overuse of sour and spicy foods, and overeating as a general problem.

The descriptive words for this type are hot, light, penetrating, pungent, intense, sharp, and acidic. Pitta controls digestion, metabolism, and energy production. The major function of this dosha is transformation.

These individuals have excellent digestion and a warmer body temperature, and they can sleep soundly for short periods of time, have an abundant array of energy, and an extraordinarily strong appetite. When disordered or imbalanced, these individuals might suffer from skin rashes, endure burning sensations, have excessive body heat, have a tendency for peptic ulcers, get heartburn, and might suffer from indigestion, too.

Pittas are powerful intellectually and they have a strong ability to concentrate well. They're overall good decision makers, speakers, and can make excellent teachers. They're exceptionally precise, sharp-witted, direct, and often desperately outspoken. They're also very ambitious and practical, and they truly love adventure and challenges. When disordered or imbalanced, these individuals can become short-tempered, highly argumentative, and suffer outbursts of emotion. When pittas feel stressed or overwhelmed, their response might be: "What did *you* do wrong?"

Pittas should follow the guidelines below:

1. Get lots of fresh air and choose cooler times of the day to get physical exercise.

2. Keep themselves cool, both physically and mentally, and apply an attitude of moderation in all areas.

3. Avoid situations of excessive heat, humidity, or steam, and ensure that plenty of fluids are consumed.

4. Be patient and considerate with others.

5. Engage in more contemplative and quieter activities.

6. Avoid situations where potential conflict could arise.

The Favorable Foods for Pitta

Pittas need cool or warm, with moderately heavy textures. They do not bide well with overly hot foods. Here, bitter, sweet, and astringent tastes are ideal for these types. They should utilize cooler, more refreshing food in summer or during the hot weather, like salads, milk, and dairy such as ice cream. Herbal teas, (specifically licorice or mint) root tea is pacifying to these individuals. Additionally, cold cereals, cinnamon toast, and apple tea are excellent breakfast ideas for pitta. Vegetarian foods work best for these individuals, as consuming red meat can heat the body from the fat content found within it. They should consume large amounts of milk, vegetables, and grains.

The Foods to Reduce for Pitta

Pittas should use less amounts of butter and added fat, and they should also avoid pickles, cheese, and sour cream, too. They should also avoid vinegar in salad dressings and use lemon juice instead. Additionally, alcoholic beverages and fermented foods should be omitted completely. The reduction of coffee intake is needed and the avoidance of oily, hot, salty, and heavier foods like fried foods. Pittas should also avoid egg yolks, hot spices, honey, nuts, and hot drinks too.

The Best Vegetables for Pitta

Bitter and sweet vegetables, like asparagus, cabbage, cauliflower, broccoli, Brussel sprouts, radishes, celery, cucumber, green beans, green peppers, leafy green vegetables, lettuce, okra, parsley, peas, potatoes, sprouts, squash, sweet potatoes, zucchini, carrot, mushrooms, and spinach.

The Vegetables in Moderation for Pitta

Eggplant, onions, hot peppers, tomatoes, chilis, and beets.

The Best Fruits for Pitta

Bananas, avocados, cherries, figs, mangoes, melons, coconuts, oranges, pineapples, plums, prunes, pears, and raisins. Fruits should be ripe and sweet, and these individuals should avoid fruits that are sour or unripe. Also avoiding oranges, green grapes, pineapple, and plums too, unless they're ripe and sweet.

The Fruits in Moderation for Pitta

Apricot, persimmon, raw papaya, sour cherries, grapefruit, berries, apples, peaches, dark grapes, and pineapples.

The Best Grains for Pitta

Barley, wheat, oats, and white rice (basmati is best).

The Grains in Moderation for Pitta

Brown rice, rye, corn, and millet.

The Best Dairy for Pitta

Butter, ghee, milk, egg whites, and fruit sorbets (not sour).

The Dairy in Moderation for Pitta

Cheese, egg yolk, sour buttermilk, sour cream, sour yogurt, and ice cream.

The Best Meats for Pitta

Chicken, turkey, shrimp, and river-caught fish (all in small amounts).

The Meats in Moderation for Pitta

Seafood and red meat.

The Best Beans for Pitta

Chickpeas, red lentils, tofu, mung beans, and other soybean products (unfermented).

The Beans in Moderation for Pitta

black lentils, black gram, and ar har dal.

The Best Oils for Pitta

Grapeseed, olive, soy, and sunflower.

The Oils in Moderation for Pitta

Almond, safflower, corn, sesame, and coconut oil.

The Best Nuts & Seeds for Pitta

Coconut, sunflower seeds, pumpkin seeds, flaxseeds.

The Best Sweeteners for Pitta

All sweeteners are acceptable, except for molasses and honey.

The Best Herbs and Spices for Pitta

Spices should generally be avoided as they are too heating for this dosha type. The following can be utilized in small amounts: mint, dill, turmeric, cardamom, cilantro (green coriander), cinnamon, coriander seed, fennel, saffron, cumin, and black pepper.

Kapha: Earth & Water

Kaphas tend to have earthy (or heavier) bodies than the other types and can store watery substances like fluids and fat more easily. They're naturally calm and attached as major characteristics. These individuals speak slowly and more melodically. They sometimes have watery-type dreams and usually have elimination that's heavy or thicker when toileting.

These individuals can be described as soft, solid, slow, heavy, steady, cold, and oily. Kapha governs the structure of the physical body. It's the principle that holds the cells together and forms the muscles, the fat, the bones, and also provides immunity. The primary function of kapha is that of protection.

Kaphas have a stronger build and have renowned stamina as well as smooth and radiant skin. They sleep soundly and have regular digestion. But when kapha go to excess they can gain weight, hold fluid, and have allergies which manifest in the physical body. When disordered or imbalanced, these individuals may become overweight, become lethargic, sleep excessively, and suffer from asthma, depression, and/or diabetes.

These individuals are naturally caring, calm, thoughtful, and loving. They have an idea or perception of general happiness, and the ability to enjoy life. They're very comfortable with routine. Kaphas are also strong, patient, loyal, steady, and supportive too. They absolutely love listening to music, enjoy reading, and they revere relaxing in a calm environment. When disordered or imbalanced, they can hold on to things including jobs and relationships. They might even do this long after they're no longer present in the moment or relationship. They can additionally display an excessive attachment style. When disordered or imbalanced, these individuals can become stubborn and resist change. When they feel stressed or overwhelmed their response is usually "I don't want to be involved."

Kaphas should follow the guidelines below:

1. Wake up earlier (before dawn), try to sleep less, and avoid sleeping during the day.

2. Get plenty of physical exercise every day.

3. Perform activities that energize and stimulate the body and the mind, as well as build the metabolic rate.

4. Allow for challenge, excitement, and a variety in life.

5. Move away from stagnation and clinging to their older ways of behavior and thought processes.

6. Keep warm and dry.

The Favorable Foods for Kapha

Warm, dry, and light food is favorable for this dosha type, or cooked (but light) meals. Kaphas fare best with lightly cooked foods or vegetables and raw fruits. Any food that's spicy is excellent for these individuals, such as very hot Mexican or Indian foods, especially during the wintertime. Dryer cooking methods (like baking, grilling, broiling, and sautéing) are best for kaphas over moist cooking like steaming, boiling, or poaching, as examples. Foods like lettuce, endive, or tonic water are great for stimulating this dosha's appetite, while their preferred spices are fenugreek, cumin, sesame seed, and turmeric.

The Foods to Reduce for Kapha

These individuals need to watch the consumption of too many fatty or sweet foods, and need to diminish their salt consumption as well, as this can lead to excessive fluid retention. They should always avoid deep-fried foods. Most individuals of this dosha have the tendency to overeat. The main meal should be at the middle of the day, and only a dry, lighter meal should be consumed in the evening. Kaphas should avoid sugar, fats, and dairy products as well, and completely avoid chilled foods and drinks, using ghee and oils in minimal amounts only.

The Best Vegetables for Kapha

Asparagus, beets, Brussel sprouts, lettuce, cabbage, broccoli, carrots, cauliflower, celery, eggplant, garlic, spinach, leafy green vegetables, lettuce, mushrooms, okra, onions, peas, peppers, radishes, and sprouts.

The Vegetables in Moderation for Kapha

Sweet potatoes, cucumbers, zucchini, and tomatoes.

The Best Fruits for Kapha

Apples, cherries, berries, cranberries, pears, apricots, papaya, prunes, pomegranates, and grapefruit. Dried fruits are good for these individuals, especially apricots, raisins, figs, and prunes.

The Fruits in Moderation for Kapha

Dates, bananas, fresh figs, coconuts, and mangoes.

The Best Grains for Kapha

Barley, corn, millet, oats, rye, buckwheat, and rice (basmati is best).

The Grains in Moderation for Kapha

Rice and wheat. Avoid hot cereals and steamed grains as they're too moist and heavy for these individuals.

The Best Dairy for Kapha

Warm skim milk, whole milk in small amounts, and eggs (not fried or cooked with butter), soy milk, goat's milk, and camel's milk.

The Dairy in Moderation for Kapha

Egg yolks.

The Best Meats for Kapha

Turkey, chicken, and lean fish (all in small amounts).

The Meats in Moderation for Kapha

Shrimp and red meat.

The Best Beans for Kapha

All legumes are acceptable.

The Beans in Moderation for Kapha

Tofu and kidney beans.

The Best Oils for Kapha

Almond, olive, sunflower, and grapeseed oil (all in small quantities).

The Best Sweeteners for Kapha

All in minute quantities.

The Best Nuts & Seeds for Kapha

Pumpkin seeds, sunflower seeds, and flaxseeds.

The Best Herbs & Spices for Kapha

All are excellent, especially cumin, sesame, fenugreek, and ginger, which is especially good for improving the digestive processes.

Chapter 4: Getting Acquainted with the Spiritual Practices as Key Elements

Ayurveda or Ayurvedic medicine is the traditional healing system of India and is often seen as a way of optimizing the proper functioning of the body. Ayurveda can assist in the healing of many conditions as well as extending an individual's life. The knowledge of Ayurveda gets its roots in the Vedas, and these are the sacred texts of India. From here, many spiritual philosophies and religions have begun. These include Buddhism, Jainism, Hinduism, yoga, and more. It's truly a science of the physical body, but it's also based upon spirituality, including the understanding of consciousness itself.

Yoga: The 'Sister' of Ayurvedic Medicine

Yoga is quite well known for its physical stretching exercises. Yoga is truly much more than this—it is a complete science and philosophy leading to enlightenment. Likewise, Ayurveda is much more than a science of understanding what foods are right for you. It is a science of using health as the basis of one's journey toward enlightenment. In fact, Ayurveda and Yoga are two sides of one coin. Ayurveda keeps the physical body healthy so that one can pursue spiritual goals, while yoga is the path of spirituality. Ayurveda is not a religion any more than yoga is a religion. They are spiritual sciences applicable to one's journey regardless of religious faith. Both sciences support a person on their journey toward self-realization or the direct knowing of their nature as spirit or soul. Scriptural study, whether it comes from the East or West, illuminates this journey.

Ayurvedic Psycho-Spirituality

The term "Ayurvedic psycho-spirituality" is based upon the idea that we all have souls which are growing and evolving toward enlightenment, which might also be called "a oneness with God" or the creator. In Ayurveda, this could be described as entering the gates of heaven. And what could be more heavenly than becoming one with God?

The 3 Gunas

The journey of our evolution is that, naturally, there are challenges which inspire us to grow and evolve, spiritually speaking. There are three gunas which form the ground which we use to understand ourselves. This occurs for individuals both emotionally and spiritually. The gunas are defined as the qualities which are found in nature.

Sattva

Sattva is the quality which represents both clarity and purity. When the mind is sattvic, or pure, there's a natural and profound connection between the individual and God. As this awareness is allowed, our most virtuous qualities can manifest. Here, the mind can be like a lake of stillness, and the light that reflects through this water is the light of God.

Rajas

Rajas is known as the state of both activity and distraction. And this is where we forget our true nature as a soul and get taken up by the dramas of our lives. As a result, individuals can get caught up in the experience of emotion, and the challenging feelings like worry, resentment, fear, anxiety, anger, and attachment. If you imagine the still lake which is sattva, rajas can be explained like a metaphor for that same lake, but during a storm. Each moving wave represents a challenging emotion.

Tamas

Tamas is the state of inertia and darkness. Here, the individual is unaware of their connection with God or the soul, but where the individual might spiral down into darkness and become harmful to the self or to others.

With the darker part being dominant, the individual might take actions such as violence or vindictive behaviors, or possibly go towards addiction or even contemplate suicide. Any harmful act reflects the individual's tamasic nature. The darkness is tamas and is the sattva lake which has become excessively toxic.

The Spiritual Journey

The spiritual journey is to move from ignorance to awareness, from dark to light, or from tamas to sattva. In Ayurvedic psycho-spirituality, the rajas and tamas are the causes of illness and/or disease. The actions which are taken, as well as the emotions felt by the rajasic and tamasic mind of the individual, push the balance of the 3 doshas, and can, therefore, lead to physical disease within the mind and/or body.

It's important to understand that sattva is the sole cause of the individual's health. Disease and/or illness will not affect the sattvic person, the individual who is awakened to the 'light.' To summarize, we could say that disease is the end result of forgetting our true nature as a soul. Once forgotten, the individual acts out of harmony with the natural flow of nature. The unbalanced actions bring about illness and/or disease. Healing involves the purposeful cultivation of balance and true harmony, or sattva.

Ayurveda & Disharmony

Ayurveda basically sees disharmony as the root cause of all illnesses and diseases. Healing takes place through a harmonious relationship with the environment within (and around) the individual.

In essence, Ayurveda prescribes many regimens to bring about harmony (sattva) in our lives. These precise regimens are numerous, and to the newcomer, can quickly seem overwhelming to practise. Some easy recommended actions include: eating slowly in a peaceful environment, using aroma and color therapy, going to bed earlier, awakening with the sunrise or before dawn, applying oil to the physical body, meditation, yoga, dietary considerations, and many more.

Many individuals ask why it's so difficult to adapt to a harmonious lifestyle. The answer is quite simple, really. It's because: when an individual isn't fully awakened to their spiritual nature, they remain unbalanced and perhaps, at times, confused about what to do within their life.

How can we live in harmony if we're not connected to our spiritual purpose in life? Without the knowledge of higher awareness, it's human nature to act as though we are only our senses, our body, and our mind. But, in truth, our senses fear what's uncomfortable and requires what gives us what might be called third dimensional pleasure or great highs. The creation of harmony within our lives brings with it a rejection of that which brings us our highs. And this is because each high is just a fleeting moment which will pass and leave us desiring more and more. And so, it really is a choice. Does the individual choose harmony or disharmony?

Ayurvedic & Yogic Practices

Ayurvedic and yogic practices can truly bring peace, and not highs. They bring energy through us; they don't burn us out. However, to get to this place, the individual must go through the 'fire' of awakening their own self-awareness.

The process of understanding the concepts of Ayurveda is honest and not always pleasurable, however. With honesty about the self, at first there's discomfort and pain, and so after this, we move away from it. Looking at the self is incredibly difficult, in fact. We must be honest and really know ourselves at this stage. We drop those practices which bring disharmony.

The Road to Empowerment

There are many roads of empowerment, but none is said to be greater than our own direct self-experience of God. This empowerment is achieved through utilizing meditation and prayer.

In the quietness of consciousness is the light of God, or what is known as "the infinite." This pure light can fill us spiritually as well as sustain us; it can empower us to create change in many areas of our lives. In truth, the more we come to know our nature as God or soul, the more we are empowered to act in harmonious ways. This process begins for many with trying the state of meditation. It ends when we meditate through every action within our lives. In essence, when our lives become a meditation, the ego self seeps away, exposing our truest nature. At this point, we're ready to join pure consciousness to pure awareness. And it is here that we are said to become one with God.

In a later chapter, we will discuss in more detail the practices related to spirituality, including meditation, yoga, and other forms of spirituality.

Chapter 5: Modern Ayurveda as a Study Base in India & Abroad

New Age Ayurveda & It's Constituents

Ayurveda has undergone true transformation over the last century, and this is because of the engagement with modernness in its various forms. The major revision of mainstream Ayurveda to fit scientific and biomedical paradigms, mostly in the Western contemporary context, has led to the recasting of this tradition, however.

Some professional scholars might even refer to the spiritualised form of Ayurveda in the West as being "New Age Ayurveda," since it displays many of the features associated with what is loosely classed as being New Age phenomena.

Ayurveda in its spiritualised form is very much a product of a move away from submission, to the external, more religious authority. From here, it has been a movement towards reliance on personal experience and in experimentation in matters which relate to faith, what is said to be sacred, as well as the questions pertaining to morality. And particularly evident in Britain's holistic health system, as an example, where practitioners have skills in a range of so-called complementary and alternative medical (CAM) traditions from different parts of the world. They can offer healing of the soul for their clientele, as well as more mainstream medicine through Ayurveda and other modalities.

Popularity for Ayurveda is Increasing

Ayurveda has gained increasing recognition within the holistic field since the 1980s, and particularly in the new millennium. Studies on New Age Ayurveda have truly tended to focus on well-established practitioners, as well as the promoters of Ayurveda in the West, and also on the popular writing authored by these individuals. There have been no formal studies which focus on examining students' engagement with Ayurvedic training programmes offered in North American and European institutions, however, or the ways in which they go on to practise Ayurveda after their completion of such courses.

Ayurveda in contemporary India, though it's central to the provision of health services nationwide, reflects the 'matrimony' of biomedicine within this subcontinent, and the Indian government's deep commitment to institutions and practices which focus on the biomedical ideals. In fact, the government has various councils and acts in place to regulate and control the practice of Ayurveda, and this helps to provide professional training, and look for standardizing an individual's education and qualifications. Additionally, the Ayurvedic institutions and colleges in India are based upon the institutional and organisational modelling which is shown in biomedicine. Ayurveda is thoroughly biomedical in the modern age.

The Standard is Being Set for a Modern Curriculum

The standardised curriculum taught at Ayurveda colleges in India are designed by a government-run body, which is the *Central Council for Indian Medicine*, which oversees the provision of Ayurvedic teaching in India. The undergraduate Ayurveda degree is the integrated *Bachelor of Ayurveda and Medical Surgery* (or BAMS).

The BAMS curriculum is organised mostly around a modern division of subjects, rather than around particular Ayurvedic texts or topics. The syllabus collaborates ancient and medieval classics, as well as multiple textbooks organised to focus upon modern times, and written in a basic textbook style, which is entirely different from the poetic or literary focus of the classical works. Additionally, it's divided up into each subject area, based upon the biomedical models as: physiology, pathology, anatomy, diagnostic techniques, pharmacodynamics, mineralogy, toxicology, pharmacology, dispensing, and internal medicine. This might vary slightly from institution to institution.

Ayurvedic theory, which traditionally doesn't make the same divisions and classifications, has been rearranged to match the biomedical theme. Also, this formalised curriculum has been separated and has no magical or ritualistic elements at all. And these had previously existed alongside therapeutic modalities but have since been said to be "primitive."

The standardised curriculum in Ayurveda also incorporates significant elements of instruction found within biomedicine, even though there's no effort to establish the elements of compatibility and/or incompatibility between the 2 differing systems. Ayurvedic subjects are taught primarily in the classrooms of colleges, and the biomedical subjects are taught mostly in laboratories and hospitals.

For entrants to both biomedical and Ayurvedic studies, and to training programmes in other branches of healthcare, students sit for a common entrance exam. In most cases, the top achievers go keenly into biomedical colleges, while others get placed into offshoots, like Ayurveda. Ayurveda clearly occupies a position of inferiority when compared to biomedicine. And students entering Ayurveda programmes are not always driven by motivation to study Ayurveda as their first choice but might simply settle for what is considered second-best after failing to make the grade for a (perceived) higher MBBS degree in biomedicine.

The students admitted to the course are coming from a Westernized system of school education, most with little to no background in Indian classical philosophy (which accentuates Ayurveda) or in Sanskrit (the language that classical texts are written in).

Many students find themselves 'drowning' in a world of Ayurvedic concepts and categories that are completely foreign to the scientific model. Students are mostly unable to acquire the familiarity with Sanskrit or the necessary time to understand the classical modes of thought and depth that would be necessary for them to comprehend the full context and depth of the principles and methods underlying Ayurveda. Ancient Ayurveda was based upon these principles.

Sometimes, Ayurvedic training in these colleges tends not to be focused adequately on the practical application of Ayurveda's methodology or principles. Some colleges aren't integrated with Ayurvedic hospitals, and so some students often assimilate theoretical concepts with little understanding of their application in real-life situations. It's also important to note that clinical training is obtained, not at Ayurvedic hospitals, but in biomedical settings, where students find themselves further removed from Ayurvedic practices. And so, unfortunately, students might get little to no exposure to India's folk traditions which can offer rich insights into local systems of the necessary knowledge related to healing and cure.

Another important factor has been that the ancient traditions have gradually fallen into disuse because of India's modern push in recent years. And so, after completing their training, many students go on to practise biomedicine using the biomedical knowledge learned in the course of their Ayurvedic training.

In many cases, Ayurveda graduates going on to set up practice as *Vaidyas* or physicians in Ayurveda, do so in clinics throughout the country of India. Ayurvedic practice remains a relatively lucrative business option in the Indian modern world.

Interestingly though, Ayurveda has a strong tradition of health maintenance and disease prevention, but Ayurvedic practice within modern India does focus mainly on its remedial aspects. And this is because the practice tends to be largely disease-oriented, where patients come in with current complaints where specific remedies are prescribed. So, because of this, Ayurveda has come to resemble the biomedical model, where the state of disease is pathologized, and health is presumed to be the "unproblematic normality." But in true, ancient Ayurveda, keeping individuals free of disease in the first place is the true goal, not using it as a 'fix' when things begin to go (or have already gone) wrong, where health is the balance.

Ayurvedic Consultations

Consultations at Ayurvedic clinics are like clinics run by general practitioners who are trained in the biomedical system. Here, the *Vaidya* examines the patient, studies any biomedical reports, including X-rays or any test results that the patient may have obtained. And then he/she writes prescriptions and, if necessary, dispenses medicines.

The medicines aren't like the traditional ones made at home from fresh herbs, and are mass-produced by pharmaceutical companies, with longer shelf-lives and (perhaps) less efficacy, in some people's opinions. The time spent on any given consultation is swifter too, so that the (usually long) queues of waiting patients can be tended to, and then patients are told to report back after a specified period of time for another consultation.

Ayurveda is now taught and practised in contemporary India, so some might say it's disconnected from its classical context, and from the ancient traditions seen in older methods of healing. And these had developed over the centuries in various parts of rural India.

Now though, Ayurveda is modelled on biomedicine in most cases, and for some, it's lacking integrity either as a traditional system and/or as a Western biomedicine. Ayurveda has come to be reinvented as symbol of so-called 'authentic' Indian tradition and culture, but many scholars and professionals state that the promoters and practitioners of Ayurveda in India are promoting Ayurveda as spiritually attuned, anti-materialistic, non-violent, and as a contrast to biomedicine. In some cases, this is true, and in some cases it's untrue.

However, interestingly, Ayurveda in the modern world takes on forms of the new, with professionalized, institutionalised practice, while also assuring the promise of deliverance to the ancient ways, which seems to be a conflict of interest for some. These modern accounts of Ayurveda are interesting to note, where India appears as a land of the more modern capabilities, as well as a traditional treasure trove of New Age wisdom, with mystical and esoteric insight, and spiritual fortitude too.

For readers of this title today, it's an important and necessary understanding that some have portrayed New Age Ayurveda as the "shallowness" and "fragility" of the "materialistic" West. In many respects, the way of modern Ayurveda training is quite lacking in the nuances from ancient times, although some practitioners promise ancient wisdom as well as biomedicine.

The Way to Ayurveda

Many embark on their Ayurvedic training after failing to make the grades required for entrance to the desired training programmes in biomedicine, as mentioned earlier, where India is concerned. But those in the United Kingdom enter their Ayurveda courses via a more complex route.

Some students described how their interest in Ayurveda was sparked by a chance encounter with a guru practitioner, who then might've have aroused their interest in them to discover more about the subject through formal study, as well as due to an interest in the more spiritual aspects of ancient Ayurveda.

In some cases, this interest was further fueled when these individuals underwent Ayurvedic treatment themselves, and so a deeper engagement with the principles underlying the system and its treatment modalities might be borne. In various other cases, the interest in Ayurveda appeared to have been triggered by the interest in (and exposure to) somewhat related systems, like yoga, meditation, or Tibetan medicine, which then led to enquiries formulating within a period, well before any formal training in Ayurveda occurred.

A couple practising in England's south coast had a journey to India that eventually led to their enrolment within the *Thames Valley Ayurveda* programme. Their trip to India occurred when they experienced disillusionment with their previous careers and lifestyles, and so they found Ayurveda.

Rachel stated,

"Ayurveda is not just about treating disease; that's just one small part really of Ayurveda. It's much more about where are you going in life, where have you come from, therefore what is your life's purpose..."

"...I read a book by Maya Tiwari, who is quite an eminent Ayurvedic healer, called Path of Practice, and it resonated very, very deeply with me actually and affected me quite a lot. I really felt deeply interested in what she was saying and

just was looking up the College on the Internet and it just kind of fell in place."

Markus described his experience below:

"I was brought up in East Germany, then when the wall came down, I went to the West of Germany and studied American literature, theater studies and American cultural studies, did an MA, and at the same time was already working at a theater. And when I finished my MA, entered into a contract as an assistant director at a theatre in Germany... I met [Rachel] backstage. Then, came a period when I realized that this is not what I want to carry on, so I started studying Shiatsu therapy and I did this for two years. I didn't finish it with a degree because we went off to India together for a year, discovered Ayurveda there, and on coming back, decided not to continue with Shiatsu but to go straight on to study Ayurveda."

When he was asked what it was that had attracted him to Ayurveda, Rohan stated,

"I think it's a personality thing with me. I have a very strong urge, and I don't know where it comes from, to really penetrate and get to the bottom of the truth of things, the truth of how things really are. I don't subscribe to the scientific model of the world because I don't believe it is a model that reflects the true nature of things, which is why I have always been interested in pursuing models of reality that include the realms of existence that are not tangible. So, that's what attracted me to astrology because its view of the world is extremely holistic. Everything has a symbolic relevance, significance that goes way beyond the reductionistic approach that science presents, in the same way that Ayurveda also has an inclusive view of the world, of the universe in fact. It's this inclusive view that attracts me

because it includes the existence of the consciousness that goes beyond embodiment."

Another graduate, Charles, who had studied with Rohan said,

"I did look at other systems, it wasn't that Ayurveda was the only system I looked at. For example, I actually went and studied hypnotherapy. I gained a qualification in that. I actually went out and studied massage as well, and reflexology, so I looked at a number of different systems that were around, and guess some of the closer systems (to Ayurveda) might have been naturopathy and things like that. I was interested in something that included some kind of spiritual and physical aspects like yoga. So, I was looking for a really complete, very holistic system. Most of the Western systems, including naturopathy which is very good, didn't include the spiritual element or the yoga element. So that really settled it for me. I was looking for a system that was totally integrated and looked at an individual human being as a complete human being. And Ayurveda was really the thing that fitted closest to that requirement for me, and that was the reason I went for Ayurveda..."

"...If we are truly spiritual beings, there is this energetic force within us and around us that we can manage actively, and that's what I do. And that's how I believe Ayurveda works ultimately. So for example in terms of food, Ayurveda looks at food from an energetic point of view rather a molecular point of view; it looks at cycles through the day from an energetic point of view rather than any other cyclical or material point of view, and also thinking processes... if that's all true then our thinking processes inherently have an energy attached to them that are capable of creating matter around us. So, all of these things paint a picture for me of a

spiritual life that means we can manage that energy in a very pro-active way."

The discovery of Ayurveda that Markus describes here was due to his chance meeting with Rajiv and Shubha Rathor, a husband and wife team, and Ayurvedic practitioners, practicing at a clinic in Mumbai.

Markus first met Rajiv in Germany at a workshop, where he got the address for the clinic. According to Rachel, Markus' wife, the Rathors belong to a lineage of physicians that dates back over 2000 years, where they're actually the twenty-second generation in an unbroken line.

Interestingly too, Rajiv Rathor's guru was Baba Gyandas Swami, a Tibetan physician living in India, under whose training Rajjiv had studied for 3 years in Mumbai. In the course of the interview with Markus and Rachel, photographs of the palm leaf scrolls handed down through successive generations of lineage were viewed, explaining that some were hundreds of years old, while others were over a thousand years old. A truly remarkable story of a journey to Ayurveda from abroad.

Here, another student who at the time of interviewing was enrolled in the Ayurveda programme at *Middlesex University*, described the spiritual basis of Ayurveda as follows:

"I think it's energy healing, isn't it? Ayurveda is energy medicine. When you talk about the herbs, you are talking about the energetics of the herbs and you are talking about the patient's energy. You are talking about the doctor's energy, you know, the energy of the equipment, the energy about the herbs. If you put it all together, it is energy healing,

so there must be something spiritual to it. Even the disease has its own energy, you know."

A Noteworthy Understanding of Energy as it Relates to the Study of Ayurvedic Medicine

Energy *can* be manipulated, and so Ayurvedic healing can be stated as the result of the ability to manage and manipulate this energy in ways conducive to an individual's personal growth and spiritual journey, and then forward to true transformation of the self.

Many individuals described Ayurveda as being "Vedic." The term carries a high symbolic value for spiritual seekers, but the term is resourceful and advocates of Ayurveda put it to multiple uses, where they attribute multiple meanings such as ancient, or divine, or timeless, or pristine, or Sanskritic, or scientific, or any of these combinations. Additionally, the term is understood to encompass, aside from Ayurveda, a very broad range of different traditions and practices including various forms of yoga and pranayama, tantra (which includes the physical body in terms of chakras), the use of mantras, yantras and mudras, pulse reading, gemology, Indian astrology, and some elements from Advaita Vedanta. All mentioned categories are perceived as parts of a complex and unified whole and are said to be completely compatible with each other and conducive to the attainment of self-knowledge or attainment.

Ayurveda is Energy, not a Category

In many ways, the terminology "Vedic field" appears as a pointer to the term "biomedicine" in modern times, especially with regards to "Ayurveda" as an umbrella term for various methods and principles which might be incorporated. But for many scholars and professionals, including Ayurvedic practitioners, biomedicine is seen to be a reductionist viewpoint, because the Vedic field is understood to be holistic and integrative, as well as scientific in its all-encompassing nature. You can't truly put it in one category therefore, for to do that is to box it up and even quash it. Energy is evermoving, and it only changes form. So, to have a completely tunnel-vision understanding of Ayurveda would be naïve according to many viewpoints on the subject.

Publications & Ayurveda

Many individuals base their understanding of Ayurveda on more of an understanding; not just from classroom lectures and prescribed readings in a syllabus, but also from other crucial sources like publications authored by popular figures. Vasant Lad, Deepak Chopra, David Frawley, and Robert Svoboda are examples.

Many of these authors promote their own spiritualised interpretations of Ayurveda to readers located within North America and throughout Europe. Some of these popular authors also visit the United Kingdom and beyond for workshop tours, lectures, to host retreats, and to offer ongoing sessions, therefore allocating students and practitioners further exposure to their ideas and worldviews.

Linkage with spirituality and yoga especially, are central to most of these popular works with regards to Ayurveda. Vasant Lad prescribes breathing exercises as well as yogic postures, mudras, and mantras, as well as astrology and gemology for removing mental and physical 'blockages,' believed to be rooted by the aggravation within doshas.

Some authors emphasize the spiritual and sacred aspects of basic human activities like eating well for wellbeing. Some might downplay Ayurveda's overriding concern with treating disease, focusing upon their own own spiritualised interpretation of Ayurvedic prescriptions relating to practices, including lifestyle and diet, and also utilizing the more ancient or mystic principles to offer their own take on what Ayurveda really is. Some might incorporate the ancient understandings and spin them off with their own spiritual reflections which are marketed to the masses for publication. Some authors might advocate a mind-body version of Ayurveda linked with quantum theory that states the importance of the mind to control and ensure health, and to enhance the individual's overall wellbeing.

Many authors state antiquity, authenticity, and true timelessness of the traditions they promote within their texts and reflections, and most popular writers on Ayurveda offer new and completely revised versions of the tradition. Some are pointed and aimed primarily at spiritual seekers within the modern Western world.

From the point of view of students of Ayurveda in modern times, these spiritual interpretations of Ayurveda hold a far greater appeal than the biomedicine versions taught within the classroom. Some individuals (who might also be students of Ayurveda) are familiar with the works of some of the authors who have been popularized in modern culture, and a large number of them may have also attended workshops and retreats led by some of the key authors who speak about their findings in a public setting. Additionally, many students of Ayurveda have personal libraries with titles by modern authors, and books by a host of other popular writers providing similarly spiritualised representations of Ayurveda's principles and practices.

Most students interviewed with relation to Ayurveda can usually understand concepts related to eternal truths and ancient wisdom, and some have hopes for their own personal and spiritual development through their engagement with Ayurveda, too. Some might also have the belief that Ayurveda provides a grand scope of multiple healing traditions, where many ideas are derived from popular representations of Ayurveda in modern times, which highlight these aspects in some way, shape, or form. And so many students go on to practising Ayurveda after obtaining their university qualifications, and their practice contains forms of Ayurveda which combine elements from the spiritualised assumptions reflected in modern texts, and the more scientific interpretations as well. We can see why practitioners may have different methodologies now.

Practising Ayurveda

After their training, most use biomedical Ayurveda and their faith in the 'Vedic field' of knowledge and forms of energy healing, where many students go on to use their skills in several different ways.

Not all degree holders set up practice as fully-fledged Ayurvedic practitioners, however, many *do* end up giving consultations, dispensing simple herbal formulations, and even provide basic massage and/or detoxification treatments for their patients.

Some set up spas and retreats to cater for all types of healing, and others offer counseling, based upon Ayurvedic knowledge, to individuals and/or groups. Some also go on to author self-help books explaining Ayurvedic principles in simpler terms. Most will offer workshops to fellow practitioners as well as everyday individuals, covering a range of subjects like Ayurvedic cookery, pulse reading, and astrology in Ayurvedic healing.

The Modern Clinics of Ayurveda

Clinics often have tastefully appointed treatment and consultation rooms. The modern practitioners usually invest a considerable amount of money in the design and décor of their consulting room/s. Decorative items, beautiful textiles, and images from South Asia, including recordings of instrumental music or chanting might be present, with soft set lighting, candles, flowers, and incense. And all these things are used to create the impression of a calmer and more relaxed retreat for consultation, far away from the individual's more stressful world.

Unlike India, practitioners spend a considerably longer length of time with patients during consultation too, explaining to them in great detail the Ayurvedic world view; offering them advice on the dietary habits and ways of being which are best related to their prakriti or constitution.

The more expensive spas and retreats' treatment packages can extend from 3 or more days, and up to a week or even a fortnight. Here, the closeness to nature, scenic beauty, and the nearness to sacred sites all promises to enhance and attune the therapeutic experience for betterment. *Vedic Health* and *Panchakarma Detox* are popular packages of choice for many clients, who enjoy their Ayurvedic experiences.

Chapter 6: Meditation, Yoga, Earthing, Chanting & Sungazing

In this chapter, we'll be discovering the 3 best meditation styles for each of the Ayurvedic doshas. To revisit your dosha type, you can go back and read the previous writing to see which one is dominant for you.

Meditation

Sometimes individuals might find it difficult to meditate, whereas other individuals wake up at the end of it, wondering where the time has gone. Meditation isn't just a quirky habit, and where Ayurveda is concerned, it's said to be the world's oldest health system and the sister science to yoga. And, according to Ayurveda, the 3 doshas are also mind types as well as body types. We already know them to be: vata, pitta and kapha. Let's see how they help with regards to meditation.

Vata is the airiest dosha; pitta is the fieriest dosha; kapha is the earthiest dosha. And the way each dosha shows up in meditation has to do with their elements.

Vatas have air-like characteristics. They're always in the mind, constantly thinking, and are highly creative and imaginative. However, sometimes this air can become excess and truly turn into a tornado of thoughts within the mind, making it almost impossible to meditate. Vatas may have some difficulty finding internal stillness because there's just so much energy moving through them all of the time.

Pittas have fire-like characteristics. They can be hyper-productive, organized, and extremely goal oriented, too. That makes sitting in meditation, when the individual is supposed to be doing nothing, exceedingly difficult for them. Pittas will try to make their meditations as productive as they can, however, and might even use the time to plan tomorrow's day or think about how they're going to move on their next project.

Kaphas have earth-like characteristics. They're exceptionally calm, grounded, and very giving, too. However, just like the earth, they can also be slower and denser. Kaphas may often turn meditation into a time for a nap. For the most part, they can't mediate lying down without falling into a deep sleep. They need a meditation that's more interactive, otherwise they won't be able to remain awake for long.

Meditation Tips for the Dosha Types

Vata:

To keep the mind focused, chanting an affirmation or mantra is key. The Sanskrit mantra "Ram," which grounds; connecting to the root chakra works very well. The affirmation "I am focused" can also help vata to stay centered within everyday life. Vatas commonly get back pain, so a meditation done in a comfortable chair can make a world of a difference during meditation.

Pitta:

For pitta, meditation will make them far more productive. Meditation has been scientifically proven to increase memory as well as brain function, and help to aid productivity and emotional wellbeing, too. Pitta should remain calm and listen to a guided meditation for best results.

Kapha:

Kaphas need to stay entertained, otherwise it's going to be nap time. A meditation using mudras is recommended. These are hand gestures that help evoke various qualities to keep the mind and body connected to each other. Moving meditations (like walking or dancing) can be wise for kaphas. Kaphas should avoid using a backrest for meditation practice too; they should remain upright so energy can flow both up and down their spine.

Meditation is Highly Beneficial for Balance

Overall, meditation is a tool to enhance the individual's life and bring the doshas back into balance. Meditation is beneficial for all 3 doshas (vata, pitta, and kapha) all year 'round. Meditation practice helps to free the mind of old, negative, and unhelpful thoughts, therefore expanding an individual's awareness and consciousness.

Some Useful Meditation Techniques

While the following 3 meditation practices can be done by anyone at any time of the year, each technique has particular qualities that are helpful for balancing a particular dosha.

Explore the qualities of these 3 practices and see which one feels right for you this season.

The Kapha Walking Meditation

During springtime, excess kapha can manifest as mental sluggishness or foggy thinking, and sometimes lethargy and a lack of motivation can occur. Ensuring helpful movement and circulation helps to prevent the heavier, thicker, damper qualities of kapha from accumulating too much. Reduce excess kapha by using meditation techniques that have opposite qualities to the dosha (e.g. lighter, livelier, more energizing ones). This meditation keeps the body moving while still enhancing focus and allowing for mental clarity.

Instructions:

1. Allow 15 to 20 minutes for practice.
2. If it's cold outside, the individual may look for a quiet place to do an indoor walking meditation, like a stretch of a hallway or a yoga area. You can utilize a part of your home if necessary.
3. Take off your shoes and socks to feel sensations more easily in the feet, and as long as your environment will allow for this.
4. Stand and pause to take a few breaths and notice how you're feeling. Set an intention for your walking meditation to feel a certain way by the end of it.
5. With a natural breath and a downward gaze, begin walking slowly and rhythmically, either in a long line or in a large circle. As you walk, you can silently use phrases as you note each step, try: Left, right, left, etc.

6. Place your mind's attention on the sole of each foot as you travel, noting the feeling as the foot lifts off the floor, moves through space, and is placed back down.
7. When you stop moving at the end of the meditation, pause to notice how you feel. Did your intention work?

The Pitta Meditation for the Breath

Pitta requires peace and quiet. The opposite of the hotter, sharper qualities of pitta. And these may increase in the mind as well as the body as the result of stress or excess heat. When excess pitta manifests as mental irritation, impatience, frustration, or perhaps anger, a meditation with cooler, more spacious qualities is needed.

Meditation using the breath redirects the intense focus of pitta. It enables it to rest on the subtle anchor of the breath. Let go of all the planning, structure, and list-making activities that often consume this dosha and make time for deep peace and quiet to reset the mind to its more tranquil state of being.

Instructions:

1. Find a comfortable chair where you won't be interrupted or have any distractions around you.
2. Sit with the spine so it's straight, resting your hands on your lap with the palms turned upwards.
3. The next step is to close your eyes; make the effort to soften the muscles of the face and jaw.
4. Place your mind's attention on the belly. And now, without controlling the breath, simply notice the natural movement and sensation of breath within the belly.

5. Do this meditation for 10 to 20 minutes, or until you feel your mind get calmer and become quieter.

The Vata Mantra Meditation

Establishing a good rhythm is one of the most effective ways to soothe an overactive mind. When the lighter, subtler, more mobile qualities of the vata dosha increase excessively due to traveling, life stresses, colder temperatures, or unsettling changes, vata often manifests as restlessness, worry, fear, depression, or anxiety. The repetition of a mantra can slow a racing mind and enhance a greater focus.

Mala beads might be helpful for tracking mantra repetitions as they have some weight to them, and the anchoring helps to balance excess vata. If you don't have mala beads, simply repeat the mantra for 5 to 15 minutes, or until you feel quiet and at peace.

Instructions:

1. Choose a mantra that works for you. This might be a single word or phrase. Use any language you like. The most important thing is that it resonates for you.
2. Sitting comfortably, close your eyes and soften the facial muscles and jaw.
3. If you have mala beads, move your thumb to move the mala beads, one bead at a time.
4. In your mind or using a whisper, repeat the mantra once for each bead, using a soothing rhythm.
5. Do this for 108 times, or until your mind feels fully focused and steadier overall.

The Art of Yoga in Ayurveda

In Western culture, true yoga practice is associated mainly with a variety of courses, including exercises for both the strengthening, and tightening of the body. In almost every locality, there are yoga centers that offer different type of yoga classes and everyone is free to choose the type of yoga that brings them the most pleasure. Ayurveda medicine became popular around 20 years ago because many individuals associated this Vedic holistic system with the prevention and treatment of various diseases through natural healing.

But How is Yoga Related to Ayurveda?

Is it true that one of the systems is primarily a healing system that focuses mainly on the health of the individual, while the other one is an Indian system for physical exercises to improve tone and help with stress reduction?

If you think this way, you might be incredibly surprised when you find out that yoga and Ayurveda are very closely related aspects of Vedic science. This is the ancient Indian philosophy of consciousness. In fact, both are ancient systems which stem from the same culture, have the same historical origins, and develop and improve when used together. Additionally, they share the same language, philosophy, and methodology, too.

It's a little difficult to designate the exact time of their formation, but if we consider the first data available from the monography the "Yoga Sutras" of Patanjali, it's around 500 BC., as the first Ayurveda treatises date was approximately 700 to 150 BC., so we can say that both Indian systems occurred at around the same time.

Ayurveda is the ancient Indian medicine, including the philosophy of which is based on a comprehensive study of the person's individuality, including the characteristics and overall connection they have with the entire world.

The name of the Vedic holistic medicine comes from Sanskrit and means the "science of life" or "the art of longevity." Ayurveda states that a person is a unique creature, integral in essence, and of the universe. Therefore, all that's inside an individual exists in the microcosm around them.

Additionally, as a science of life, Ayurveda is not just a glorified medical system that treats diseases, in fact, it's a science of the right way of life which is aimed at achieving optimal health, longevity, and youth. This holistic system is geared to heal, leads individuals on the path to self-realization, and allows for the unlocking of vital energy.

In Ayurveda, the health of a person (including the mind and spiritual aspects) develops together. Because it's not enough just to be alive, you have to have higher goals and aspirations that will make your life valuable as well as meaningful. Ayurveda defines wellbeing as the harmony of the body, the mind, and the higher self. It's this drive to the higher self which connects this science to yoga.

Let's Discover Yoga

Yoga relates to the consciousness as the individual's main center. This is a science and is the main goal where the individual strives to reach pure consciousness, internal harmony, and overall bliss.

Yoga comes from Sanskrit and means "union" and "unity." In fact, it's not only a path from the physical aspect to the spiritual, but it's a union between the individual and universal consciousness into oneness. It balances both the mind and body by gradually allowing the person to rediscover their full potential, psychologically, physically, and spiritually speaking.

Yoga is both a mind and body practice. It has a renowned 5000-year-old history in ancient Indian philosophy.

There are various styles of yoga which combine breath work, physical postures, and meditation or relaxation. More recently it has become popular worldwide, and as a form of physical exercise which is mostly based upon poses which promote the improved control of the mind and body to enhance an individual's overall wellbeing.

There are different types of yoga and many disciplines within the ancient and revered practice. Here, we'll take a closer look at the history, philosophy, and various branches of yoga. We'll also take a look at some of the types of yoga used in the modern world.

It's true too, that in modern times, yoga has expanded to all corners of the globe. While it is now a popular form of exercise and a form of movement meditation, this has not always been the case.

The History of Yoga

There's no actual written record for the true inventor of yoga. Male yoga practitioners are known as yogis, and female yoga practitioners are known as yoginis. Both males and females practiced and taught yoga well before any written account of yoga came into existence.

The art was more practiced by males at first, and so, the yogis passed the discipline down to their well-disciplined students, and further down the line. After this, many different schools of yoga developed as the practice expanded its worldwide reach and popularity that we see in various localities today.

The "Yoga Sutra," is a 2,000-year-old treatise on yogic philosophy. It was made by the Indian sage known as Patanjali. This guidebook on how to master the mind, control the emotions, and grow spiritually is a popular manifestation for those who enjoy yoga. The *Yoga Sutra* is the earliest record of yoga, which was written as a guide and is one of the oldest texts in existence. It generally provides the framework for all modern yoga that we see today.

Yoga is more thoroughly known for its postures and poses, but they weren't a key part of the ancient yoga traditions in India. In fact, the individual's fitness wasn't the ultimate goal. And instead, practitioners and followers of yogic tradition focused upon other practices, such as expanding spiritual energy using breath work and using mental focus as a key element or tool.

Overall, the tradition began to gain most of its popularity in the West at the end of the 19th century. An array of interest in postural yoga occurred as early as the 1920s and 1930s, first in India and later in the thirsty Western world.

The Yoga Philosophy

To portray its bigger spiritual message and guide sessions, yoga utilizes the imagery of a tree with roots, including a trunk, its branches, the blossoms, and its fruits. Each "branch" of yoga signifies a different focus and set of characteristics.

The 6 Branches:

1. Hatha yoga: The physical and mental branch which is well-designed to prime the body and mind.
2. Raja yoga: The branch which involves meditation and strict cohesion to a series of disciplinary steps known to be the "8 limbs" of yoga.
3. Karma yoga: The path of service that aims to create a future which is free from negativity and free from selfishness.
4. Bhakti yoga: The path of devotion, a positive way to channel emotions and cultivate both acceptance and tolerance.
5. Jnana yoga: The path of yoga related to wisdom, and the path of the scholar; developing the intellect through study.
6. Tantra yoga: The path of ritual, ceremony, or the consummation of a relationship.

Approaching yoga with a specific goal in mind can help the individual to decide which branch to follow. Some follow more than one path within their lifetime.

The Importance of the Chakras

The word we know as "chakra" literally means "spinning wheel."

Interestingly, yoga acknowledges that the chakras are the center points of energy, of the thoughts, the feelings, and of the physical body which is made up of flesh and bone. According to most yogic teachers, the chakras can change the way people experience their own reality via their emotional reactions, desires or aversions, levels of confidence or fear, and via the physical symptoms and effects of these symptoms into illness/es and/or disease/s.

When the chakra energy becomes blocked, it is said to trigger physical, mental, or emotional imbalances. The symptoms can be seen and manifest as poor digestion, anxiety, depression, lethargy, and many other ailments too.

Asanas & Yoga

Asanas are the physical positions seen within the practice of Hatha yoga. Individuals who practice yoga use asanas to free up their energy and to stimulate an imbalanced chakra.

The 7 Chakras:
1. Sahasrara
   This is the "thousand-petaled" or "crown" chakra and it represents the state of pure consciousness. This is located at the crown of the head. The color white or violet represents it. Sahasrara relates to inner wisdom and physical death.
2. Ajna

This is the "command" or "third-eye chakra" and its where 2 important energetic streams in the body meet up. Ajna is associated with the colors of violet, deep blue, or indigo, although traditional yoga practitioners describe it as being primarily white. The ajna chakra is associated with the pituitary gland which pushes forth as growth and development.

3. Vishuddha

This is the "especially pure" or "throat" chakra. Red or blue are the colors associated with vishuddha. Practitioners consider this chakra to be the place of speech, of metabolism, and of hearing.

4. Anahata

This is the "unstruck" or "heart" chakra, and it's associated with the colors green and pink. Key factors involving anahata include the more complex emotions, like tenderness, compassion, unconditional love, rejection, equilibrium (or balance), and wellbeing.

5. Manipura

This is the "jewel city" or "navel" or "solar plexus" chakra. Yellow is the color associated with this chakra. Practitioners connect this chakra to personal power, the digestive system, fear, anxiety, developing opinions, and to the tendencies of having an introverted personality.

6. Svadhishthana

This is the "one's own base" or "pelvic" or "sacral" chakra. This chakra is associated with the color orange and it's primarily linked to the reproductive organs, the adrenal gland, and to the genitourinary system.

7. Muladhara

This is the "root support" or "root chakra" and it's located at the base of the spine in the coccygeal area. This primal chakra is linked to our natural urges associated with food, sex, sleep, and survival, as well as being linked to the individual's source of fear and avoidance.

Modern Yoga

Modern yoga has really been more concerned with a focus on strength, physical exercise, breathing, and flexibility. It can really help to boost an individual's physical and mental wellbeing.

There are many types of yoga, and no style is more authentic or superior to any other. The main goal is to choose a class that's appropriate for your fitness level or goals. Some of the more advanced techniques can take months (or even years) of practice to perform.

Ashtanga Yoga

This type of yoga uses the principles of ancient yoga teachings. It truly became popular during the 1970s. Ashtanga uses 6 established sequences of postures that link every movement to breath work.

Bikram Yoga

Sometimes known as "hot" yoga, Bikram yoga is done in artificially heated rooms at temperatures of nearly 105 degrees with 40 to 50 percent humidity. It's made up of 26 poses and a sequence of 2 breathing exercises.

Hatha Yoga

This is a general term for any type of yoga that teaches the physical postures. Hatha classes usually help as the introduction to the basic yoga postures.

Iyengar Yoga

This yoga focuses on finding the truest alignment in each pose by using a range of props, like blocks, straps, blankets, chairs, bolsters, and more.

Jivamukti Yoga

Jivamukti yoga translates to "liberation while living." This yoga emerged in 1984 and includes spiritual teachings and practices that are based on the fast-paced flow between poses, and not on the poses themselves.

This main focus here is called "vinyasa." Each class has a particular theme that's explored through chanting, meditation, yoga scripture, asana, music, and pranayama. Jivamukti yoga can be very physically intense.

Kripalu Yoga

This type of yoga teaches the student how to accept, know, and to learn from the physical body. A student learns to find their own level of practice by looking inwardly, in fact. The classes mostly begin with breathing exercises and gentler-type stretches, and then a series of individual poses ensue after that, followed by a final relaxation.

Kundalini Yoga

Kundalini literally means "coiled like a snake." Kundalini yoga is an ancient system of meditation that helps the individual to release built-up energy.

A class for kundalini usually begins with chanting and ends with some productive singing. In the middle of the chanting and singing, there may be features of asana, pranayama, and meditation which is relevant to creating a specific outcome.

Power Yoga

Created in the late 1980s, practitioners designed this active and athletic type of yoga which was based on the traditional ashtanga system.

Sivananda Yoga

This yoga is system based upon a 5-point philosophy. This philosophy states that relaxation, diet, proper breathing, exercise, and positive thoughts work together to form a healthy yogic lifestyle. In most cases, it uses the same 12 basic asanas, finished with some sun salutations and savasana poses.

Viniyoga Yoga

Viniyoga yoga can be adapted to any individual, regardless of their physical capabilities. Viniyoga teachers tend to be experts with regards to anatomy and yoga therapy. Many of them have studied for years before teaching classes, in fact.

Yin Yoga or Taoist Yoga

This is a meditative and quiet yoga practice. Yin yoga allows the release of tension in the key joints, including: the knees, the ankles, the hips, the entire back, the neck, and the shoulders, too.

The yin poses are passive, and this means that gravity allows most of the force and effort which is not always the case in other types of yoga.

Prenatal Yoga

Prenatal yoga utilizes postures that have been designed for women who are pregnant. It can support individuals in getting back into shape after pregnancy, too. It was primarily designed to support women during pregnancy as a lighter way of exercising and meditating.

Restorative Yoga

This is a truly relaxing version of yoga. An individual spends a restorative yoga class in 4 or 5 easy-to-do poses, using aides like blankets and bolsters to enable deep relaxation without exerting any effort while holding the pose.

The Intrinsic Connection Between Yoga and Ayurveda

The basis of Yoga is Ayurveda, and the fruit of Ayurveda is yoga...

According to ancient legend, the knowledge of these 2 systems was given by the Gods to the ancient Indian sages, and then it was given to the people. Both traditions (Ayurveda and yoga) are unique in and of themselves, and this is because of their harmony and honesty, beauty, and greatness which isn't seen within any other culture.

The goal of yoga and Ayurveda is to help the individual to take care of their own wellbeing. We might even call Ayurveda "yogic medicine" because it follows a yogic approach towards healing. The yoga system is a science of self-realization and is the ultimate goal of Ayurveda as a science of life.

In Ancient India, these 2 practices of the Vedic science didn't exist in separation. Yoga was taught only after the student understood the Ayurvedic principles, however. This was because, it was only allowed *after* the development of the physical component of health was achieved, and when the person was healthy. Therefore, the individual could go on to achieve emotional balance and spirituality.

Ayurveda gives the basis for the health and wellbeing of the body and mind by allowing for the right diet, additional herbs, prime exercises, the use of massages, and other lifestyle factors. Yoga teaches individuals how to develop higher consciousness through various methods, including asanas, pranayama, and via meditation practices.

The Human Being is More

The human being is not only a physical body or a set of biochemical processes occurring within flesh. Instead, the human being is a complex makeup of physical parts, with a soul and a mind, and where the ego resides. This is why the real potential is not only physical, but psychological, spiritual, and emotional. We need realization at all these vital levels.

While the physical body is the general foundation, spirituality is the ultimate goal, and the mind is the main tool for development. Utilizing a healthy system that affects human nature in a complex way is what occurs with yoga and Ayurveda as a complementary set of healing practices.

We could say, yoga and Ayurveda are connected by a common cultural and historical origin, and together they form the overall understanding of health and the achievement of self, including the awareness and consciousness of the individual.

Within Ayurveda, by identifying the prakriti (or constitution) of an individual, this allows the choice of the right yoga practices for the individual. These may be asanas, cleansing techniques, meditation, and the harmonization of yoga practice according to the individual's biorhythms and seasons.

In essence, yoga practice allows a way to cleanse the spirit, and it includes spiritual self-realization. So, in truth, it's said that one system can't function without the other, because they're the 2 parts of the same whole. Each one of these disciplines has its own unique place and function, and each of them overlaps with the other at differing levels.

The Similarities Between Yoga & Ayurveda

1. Both practices recognize that maintaining a healthy body is vital for the implementation of the 4 main goals in each person's life: Dharma, Arta, Kama, and Moksha.

112

2. Both practices believe that balancing the doshas is of great importance to maintain good health and wellbeing.
3. Both practices believe that a balanced eating regime must be followed, and the use of herbs, meditation, asanas, pranayama, mantras, and practices that heal the body, mind, and spirit are necessary.
4. For both practices, good health is the basis of psychological, emotional, and spiritual wellbeing as a triune necessity.
5. Both practices use methodologies to cleanse the body and that can stimulate the natural detoxification of the individual, by following natural routes of expulsion. In Ayurveda, the Panchakarma procedure (5 cleansing actions) is applied, and for yoga the procedure is called Shat Karma (6 actions).
6. Both practices have almost the same physiology and anatomy, and these consist of 72, 000 fine channels (nadi), 7 main energy centers (chakras), 5 body shells, and energy (kundalini shakti).
7. Both practices have the 5 basic elements present (air, earth, ether, water, fire).

The Differences Between Yoga & Ayurveda

Despite the existing similarities, there are some minute differences between the 2 sciences.

1. Ayurveda provides for the balance of body and mind by using all that nature provides, including plants, stones, fragrances, water, and air.

2. Yoga helps to harmonize the consciousness and the physical body using special techniques such as prayers with certain sounds, asanas, breathing practices

(pranayama), and different types of meditation techniques.

3. Ayurveda seems to be more medical or science-based, whereas yoga is more spiritual based and aimed at the liberation from suffering.

Even though the 2 complementary practices have little differences in their approaches, both yoga and Ayurveda have one ultimate goal, which is to help the individual to reach a higher level of self-awareness and to achieve great health.

Yoga, Ayurveda & Prana

Prana connects the individual to the body and the mind. It also connects Ayurveda and yoga practices which are concerned with both. Prana or "the power of life" is a manifestation of the divine powers. It's also true that Vedic philosophy, the full healing and transformation of the individual, is accomplished through prana, which ultimately is known to be "the power of the spirit."

Interestingly too, everything that we perceive (food, impressions, and breath,) is a means for prana. And so, prana connects us with our higher self.

Yoga brings the individual to calmness and balance, and the yogic exercises have protective and healing functionalities too. And although most people associate yoga with the physical exercises, its focus is truly on improving the spirit, the mind, and the body.

Yoga practice helps with the implementation of the natural order and balance in metabolic and hormonal levels. It improves metabolism, and helps to alleviate the diseases related to it, such as hypertension, diabetes, asthma, and obesity.

The Ultimate Goal

Ayurveda and yoga are 2 complementary practices and are linked parts of an ancient Vedic science. Both systems are purpose-filled towards the goal to make our lives better and more valuable, showing the individual how to understand their true nature. This filters out and aids the individual further, by enabling the individual to make the right choices and to undertake the proper measures to be healthier, happier, and to achieve spiritual peace and calm both within, and with the world that surrounds them.

The path of yoga and Ayurveda are symbiotic, in that one without the other would mean that something is missing. They are equal parts to a greater whole, incorporating the essence of ancient wisdom together, where each practice benefits the other in a complementary manner.

What is Earthing & Why is it Important?

Environmental medicine primarily addresses environmental factors which have a negative impact on an individual's health. Additionally, scientific research has revealed a surprisingly positive and vastly negated environmental factor on health. And so, this is the direct contact with the immeasurable supply of electrons on the surface of the planet.

Modern lifestyle can move people away from such contact. The research suggests that this disconnect may come forth as illness eventually, especially when mixed with other toxic lifestyle factors. In fact, the reconnection with the planet's electrons has been found to promote intriguing physiological changes as well as positive and subjective reports of wellness.

Earthing (also known as grounding) incorporates many benefits including better sleep and reduced pain. It can be achieved from sitting or walking outside barefoot, while working, or even sleeping inside while connected to systems of conductivity that transfer the planet's grounding electrons from Earth's surface and into the body.

It's true to say that environmental medicine looks at the interactions between an individual's health and to the environment, including factors which include air and water, and toxic chemicals which compromise health. It's also true that environmental medicine focuses upon how these factors cause or mediate illness and disease, too.

We could say that the one factor which is present throughout the environment is surprisingly beneficial, yet mostly overlooked as a prime resource for health maintenance, including illness and disease prevention, as well as within clinical therapy.

The actual surface of the earth possesses a non-limited and continuously renewable supply of free and mobile electrons. This surface is uniquely and electrically conductive (except in the driest places, like deserts), and its negative potential is always applicable, and this is because the electron supply is constantly replenished by the atmospheric electrical circuit on a global scale.

The Earth's negative potential can potentially (according to science) create a stable bioelectrical environment which is internal, and this could allow for the normal functioning of all body systems. Additionally, the research extends to being able to maintain an individual's setting of their biological clock and also regulating body rhythms.

Additionally, the electrons from molecules (which are antioxidant) neutralize reactive oxygen species (ROS, or free radicals) and these are part of the body's immune and inflammatory responses.

Both Western science and Ayurvedic science point to the same assumptions, and many scientific studies have shown that there's the potential that the influx of free electrons absorbed into the body through direct contact with the ground, will most likely neutralize the free radicals and help to reduce chronic inflammation and/or acute inflammation found within the individual's body.

In ancient times, dating back thousands of years, humans primarily walked barefoot or had shoes made from animal skins. They also slept on the ground or on top of these animal skins. This direct contact (or via sweat-moistened animal skins used as shoes or sleeping mats) utilized the ground's unending free electrons. And so, were able to enter the physical body, which is, as we know, a thorough conductor of electricity. Via this mechanism of action, every part of the physical body could harmonize (at an equilibrium) with the electrical potential of the ground, and stabilize the electrical environment of all cells, tissues, and organs.

Modern Lifestyle Impacts

Modern lifestyle has increasingly separated human beings from the vastness of flow of Earth's electrons. And since the 1960s to 70s, we have increasingly worn rubber or plastic-soled shoes which insulate, instead of the leather-fashioned-type shoes made from animal hides. In essence, this has separated us from the grounding of the earth's energy field, and we rarely sleep on (or near) the ground, either.

In recent times, immune disorders, chronic illness, and inflammatory diseases have increased rapidly, and some researchers have stated that the modernness of newer environmental factors are the cause. And due to the disconnection with the earth's surface, this, as a cause, has rarely been brought to the fore, although many research papers suggest a trend in that direction.

A Natural Approach

It was in the late 19th century when Germany claimed more of a natural approach, utilizing health benefits from being barefoot outdoors, and even doing so in colder weather. A modern doctor (White) looked into the practice of sleeping grounded in his research, and did so after being told by some that they couldn't sleep properly "...unless they were on the ground or connected to the ground in some way." For some, the use of copper wires attached to and grounded-to-Earth gas, water, or radiator pipes worked for these individuals. The doctor also reported improved sleep using these differing techniques, but his ideas never caught on in mainstream society during that time of research.

Experimentation in Poland revealed succinct physiological and beneficial health benefits with the use of bed pads, mats, EKG and TENS-type electrode patches which were conductive, and also with plates connected inside to the earth outside.

A retired cable television executive (Ober) found a closeness between the human body and the cable used to transmit television signals via cable. He noticed that when cables are "grounded" to the earth, any meddling is virtually eliminated from the signal. Additionally, all electrical systems are stabilized by grounding them to the earth.

Others discovered that grounding the human body represented a "universal regulating factor in nature," which strongly influenced the bioelectrical, bioenergetic, and biochemical processes, overall. The studies also appeared to offer an impactful and modulating effect where chronic illnesses were shown.

Earthing Systems Have Even Been Patented

Earthing is also known as "grounding" and really refers to contact with Earth's surface electrons. So, by walking barefoot outside or working, sitting, or sleeping indoors while connected to conductive systems, an individual can benefit. And some of these conductive systems have been patented, and work to transfer the energy from the ground into the physical body. Interestingly too, much scientific research supports the concept that the planet's electrons induce an endless array of physiological changes of notable significance, including reduced pain, better sleep patterning, the shift from sympathetic to parasympathetic tonality in the autonomic nervous system (ANS), and even ensuing a blood-thinning effect. The research, along with many anecdotal reports, are in line with Ayurvedic medicine and its naturally based approach.

Helping Your Dosha with Earthing

How can walking barefoot help balance your dosha?

Walking barefoot on any surface which is natural lets individuals connect directly to the earth and its magnetic field. It's believed (and shown through science) that the relationship between our physical bodies and Earth's natural electrons is significant, providing us with a plethora of notable health benefits. Scientific studies report a significant difference in the regulation of the body's nervous systems, helping to reduce stress, while also reducing inflammation, increasing antioxidants, and allowing improved sleep.

In Ayurveda Earthing is a Natural Implementation

In Ayurveda, it's believed that individuals are made up with energies of the 5 great elements. These are: space, air, fire, water, and earth. These can manifest in doshas, and we already know these to be vata, pitta, and kapha. We're all made up of a unique combination of these 3 forces. When unbalanced, nature can have an impact on balancing these energies.

Overall, earthing can bring an abundant amount of health benefits to an individual's life. However, for every individual, the health benefits may differ, depending upon their dominant dosha.

Vata Earthing

Vata is definitely the most fragile of the 3 doshas, and the individual can fall out of balance quite quickly. As a vata, sometimes the individual may feel ungrounded and have a mind which is racing with clear signs of excessive air and wind. This is an important time to seek out the stability of the groundedness of the earth.

Vatas might even begin to lean toward the long and slim figure with thin skin and a natural coldness of the body that comes on quickly and seems to vibrate throughout their system. When earthing, these individuals should try to choose a warm environment as well as a softer surface, where possible. Vatas naturally embody the qualities of hardness, so walking on hard surfaces may increase their sense of rigidness.

It can also be important not to make their body temperature even colder. To balance the cold nature of vata, spending a little time in the sun, allowing its light and warmth to penetrate, is vital. In these moments, the vata individual can reflect upon the life and energy-giving force of the sun and allow it to warm and regenerate them.

Pitta Earthing

With an excess of pitta, it's easy to feel overheated and very irritable. Earthing in these times can be important to help balance the fire out, and to see things with more clarity.

Pitta does exceptionally well from the cooler and moister environments. Walking in the hot summer (for example) would make it unattractive for pitta types and so it would be far better to walk in the water alongside the shoreline of a beach. Allowing the water's cooling influence to calm and soothe pitta is key.

To aide with any anger or digestion issues, surrounding these individuals with luscious vegetation, the color of green plants, the blue sky, and the richness of the ground's earth is excellent. These are especially pacifying for this dosha.

Walking in the morning dew on the grass can help in boosting immunity, and in cooling the physical body. This also helps to ease inflammatory conditions for pitta. Additionally, the moon during the night-time has an immense cooling influence and is very soothing to this dosha type.

Kapha Earthing

Kapha can get through exceptionally difficult terrain and is the most tolerable to the ground conditions while earthing. With excessive kapha, it's common to feel dull and overly lethargic traits, sometimes with a lack of energy and motivation. In these moments, these individuals should seek out the elements of space and air and get outdoors as much as possible.

The more kaphas move, the more energy is created within their physical body, resulting in a burst and a boost of energy. Moving the muscles and increasing circulation is also highly advantageous for these types.

The best experience with air is the breath. In fact, taking a few deep breaths when earthing will allow for the full-body experience and also allows kapha to reap the benefits of the experience.

Kaphas do best choosing to walk on tough terrain with different-shaped stones and sticks. The differing textures beneath their feet will invigorate them and increase the circulation even more so.

What is Chanting?

Mantras are sacred sounds that are known to impact our frequency, vibration, and energy at a cellular level, and truly offer a vital role in healing the physical body, the mind, and the spirit.

Mantras are often chanted in Sanskrit. They are believed to have spiritual and psychological powers that work on the level of one's consciousness. They can really be vital in the overall healing process, too.

In Ayurveda, mantras are often used to balance the doshas. When using mantras with functional Ayurvedic wisdom to balance the doshas, the chants can act as a real shift for healing, general wellness, and overcoming subconscious blocks in the nadis and chakras (or subtle body).

The mantras are also a significant part of the individual's spiritual practice. Mantras can be chanted out loud or adhered to silently, and they're often chanted 108 times with a mala.

The Benefits of Chanting

1. Can be soothing to the physical body and mind, working at a consciousness and on a cellular level.
2. Releases negative thought patterns and overthinking.
3. Can reduce depression, anxiety, and lift one's emotional mood.
4. Incorporates compassion and connects to the love energy (or bhakti).
5. Supports wellness, immunity, and balances the doshas.
6. Aids intuition and divine guidance.
7. Is free and easy to do.
8. Increases magnetism and radiance.
9. Clears the throat chakra.
10. Helps with meditation and improves mental focus.

Balancing the Vata Dosha

To bring balance to vata, the individual may add chants and mantras that vibrate more earth and water energy. A warming energy is also highly conducive and balancing.

Some symptoms which may be present when the vata dosha is out of balance are anxiety, worry, overwhelm, ungroundedness, inability to focus and finish projects, nervous system disorders, rapid or rambling speech, feeling cold, feeling excessive dryness, gas, constipation, alternating constipation, and diarrhea.

For the most part, anytime there's change or inconsistency resulting in movement in the mind and body, vata will become unbalanced.

Using sounds that are warmer, more grounding, more soothing, gentler, calmer, slower, sweeter, and more rhythmical are best.

> **Basic Chants for Vata** (_pronunciation_ in _parentheses following the term)._
>
> Vam (pron. Vum), Lam (pron. Lum), Gam (pron. Gum), Klim (pron. Kleem), Shrim (pron. Shreem), Hrim (pron. Hreem).
>
> Om (pron. Aum), Klim (pron. Kleem), Shrim (pron. Shreem), Hrim (pron. Hreem), Namaha.
>
> Vam (pron. Vum), Lam (pron. Lum), Om (pron. Aum).

Additional Chants:

> _Invocation to Ganesha_
>
> Pronunciation: Om Gam Ganapataye Namah
>
> Meaning: Salutations to Ganesha. Grant me freedom from obstacles.
>
> Ganesha is said to be the god of success, wisdom, and the remover of obstacles.

Adi Mantra (Gurmukhi Mantra)

<u>Pronunciation:</u> Oong Namo Gurudav Namo

Meaning: I bow to the creative energy of the infinite. I bow to the divine channel of wisdom.

This mantra opens the communication channels between the divine teacher and the learning student, and also opens the student up to new endeavors, and gives them the necessary strength to try something different or new.

The mantras work well when repeated throughout the day and before (or after) meditation practice. They may be repeated 108 times or in any denomination borne from that number.

Balancing the Pitta Dosha

This dosha is made mainly from fire and a little water, so, to bring balance to this dosha, the individual may add chants and mantras that vibrate with the cooler energy of the earth, water, and with the air element, or with love.

Some unwanted symptoms that appear when this dosha is unbalanced are anger, blame, criticism, feeling hot, intense and excessive focus which can lead to burnout, sharpness in speech, diarrhea, rashes, heartburn (acid reflux), and inflammation of any type within the physical body. Overall, whenever there's too much heat and intensity in the mind and physical body, pitta will become aggravated.

Sounds that are cooler, that soothe the mind, which are calmer, gentler, slower, sweeter, and more rhythmical work well.

Basic Chants for Pitta

Vam (pron. Vum), Lam (pron. Lum), Yam (pron. Yum), Shrim (pron. Shreem), Aim.

Om (pron. Aum), Shrim (pron. Shreem), Aim, Namaha.

Vam (pron. Vum), Lam (pron. Lum), Om (pron. Aum).

Additional Chants:

Shant Mantra

Pronunciation: Om (pron. Aum) Santih Santih Santih O-M (pron. A-U-M) Shanti Shanti Shanti

Meaning: Om Peace Peace Peace

More Advanced Shant Mantra

Pronunciation: Sarveshamsvastir Bhavatu Sarveshamshantir Bhavatu Sarveshampurnam Bhavatu Sarveshammangalambhavatu.

Meaning: May there be well-being for all, may there be peace for all. May there be wholeness for all, may there be happiness for all.

Increases peace and wellbeing for individuals who say it.

So Hum (or Silent Breath Meditation) by Dr. Vasant Lad

"When sound, breath, and awareness come together, it becomes light... So, Hum meditation properly practiced leads to the union of the individual with the universal Cosmic Consciousness. You will go beyond thought, beyond time and space, beyond cause and effect. Limitations will vanish." - *Dr. Vasant Lad*

The *So Hum Meditation* has existed in India throughout the millennia. It joins the movement of the breath with the mantra which fits easily and naturally into the inhalation (So) and to the exhalation (Hum). "So" is both felt and said mentally during the whole phase of inhalation, and "Hum" occurs during the exhalation of the breath.

The meaning of "So Hum" is "I am that" while the deeper meaning of the translation is translated to "I am that pure awareness." The mantra was made to completely calm the mind, and it also simultaneously focuses it as well as sharpens it to advancing clarity.

Instructions for the So Hum Silent Breath Meditation

1. Begin by taking some slow, deep breaths, establishing the practice of a fuller breath. When you are ready to practice So Hum, you can move your awareness when ready.

2. As you breathe inwardly, feel the inhalation at the base of the spine, or the root. With the inhale, bring your awareness up to the front of the body, along the middle, and then to the center of the brain. In your mind you chant "So" during this inhalation breath. When you reach the end of the inhale, hold the breath for a short time.

3. Next, and as you breathe out, silently (in your mind) chant "Hum." You can now visualize the

128

breath leaving the center of the brainstem, and see it in your imagination as moving down the throat and returning to the base of the spine along the middle of the back of the physical body. When you reach the end of the exhale, pause before beginning again.

Mantra Therapy for Balancing the Kapha Dosha

The kapha dosha consists of earth and water, so to bring balance to kapha, the individual may add chants and mantras that vibrate with airier and ether-type energies.

Some symptoms that might occur when this dosha is out of balance are increased stubbornness, melancholy, congestion, depression, dullness, unchangeability, slower digestion, nausea, sleepiness after meals, water retention, weight gain, and becoming overly attached to possessions and/or people. Additionally, and with the lack of physical movement, dullness, and/or too much moisture and sweetness, kapha will become unbalanced. An example might be getting allergies in the springtime.

Sounds should be warming, inspiring, invigorating, uplifting, slower, sweeter, and more rhythmical.

Basic Chants for Kapha

"By intensive awareness of one's identity with the Highest Reality enshrined in a mantra and thus becoming identical with that Reality, the mind itself becomes mantra." - Shiva Sutra II

Ram (pron. Rum), Yam (pron. Yum), Ham (pron. Hum), Om (pron. Aum), Hrim (pron. Hreem), Shrim (pron. Shreem).

Om (pron. Aum), Aim, Hrim (pron. Hreem), Shrim (pron. Shreem), Namaha.

Rum, Yum, Ham (pron. Hum), Om (pron. Aum)

Additional Chants:

Sat Nam

Pronunciation: Saaaaaaat Nam

> Here, the word "Sat" is extended 8 times longer than the word "Nam." You can radiate from the base of your spine to the center of your head, and to do this, you may make the "Sat" 30-40 times longer than the "Nam."

Meaning: Truth is my name.

This mantra is used primarily in the kundalini yoga practice, where Sat Nam can be an interesting way to tune the individual's intuition.

This mantra can be repeated out loud throughout the day and before (or after) meditation. It's also great to combine breathwork and chanting for kapha.

Chants for the 3 Doshas: Vata, Pitta, & Kapha

Here are some lengthier mantras which may be used for overall healing, and these are excellent for all 3 doshas.

Gayatri Mantra

<u>Pronunciation</u>: Om Bhur Bhuvah Svah Tat Savitur Varenyam Bhargo Devasya Dhimahi Dhiyo Yo Nah Prachodayat.

Meaning: Earth, heaven, and the whole between, the excellent divine power of the sun. May we contemplate the radiance of that god, may this inspire our understanding.

This mantra is one of the oldest in Sanskrit. It speaks about the unity of all creation, even though it has many forms. Chanting calls upon the light of the sun and helps individuals to transcend any kind of suffering.

Mahamrtyunjaya Mantra

<u>Pronunciation</u>: O-M (<u>pron.</u> A-U-M) Tryambakam Yajamahe Sugandhim Pushti-Vardhanam Urvarukamiva Bandhanan Mrityor Mukshiya Mamritat.

This mantra restores both health and happiness and brings true calmness in the face of death. When determination or courage feel like they're blocked up, it helps the individual to overcome obstacles. It's also said to awaken a healing force that reaches deep into the psyche of the mind, filtering into the physical body as well.

The mantra attracts positivity, and this energy creates an inner environment to enhance the effectiveness of whatever might be taken to heal the body. And so, this mantra can be used whenever any restorative process is undertaken by the individual. The mantra can, therefore, be recited when taking medicines, as it helps to prepare the body and mind to make the best use of them. Additionally, in India, whenever matters of vitality, health, nurture, or freedom from the fear associated with death arise, this mantra is used as a remedy and as a comfort.

It's a great mantra for healing professions too, as they can benefit from reciting the mantra regularly. It's said that for practitioners who do so, they can inevitably draw from infinite reserves of energy, and also prevent burnout while opening a channel of healing from where life can be nourished.

Om Namah Shivaya

According to the Vedas, this chant allows for deep spiritual experiences and even supernatural gifts, and this is especially true when it's practiced with skill and devotion to its meaning.

Pronunciation: Om (pron. Aum), Namah, Shivaya.

Meaning: Before there was a universe, there was a vibrationless void of pure existence. Out of this void came the vibration which started the universe, which is known as "Om." The next part of the meaning is "to bow" and is followed by the word "Shivaya" which translates to "Shiva" and means "the inner divine self."

There is a deeper meaning too, and according to Shaivism, when understood intrinsically it means "I bow to the inner self."

The repeated manta 108 times works well, and while the individual visualizes themselves bowing to their true inner self. The regular practice of this mantra with focus is said to support one's understanding and awakening of the divine self within.

Siri Gayatri Mantra

Pronunciation: Ra Ma Da Sa Sa Say So Hung

Meaning: Sun, moon, Earth, infinity. All that is in infinity, I am thee.

This is a chanted meditation to send restoring and healing energy to the self, and to other individuals who may need it when necessary. When practicing kundalini yoga, the pose for this meditation is just as important as the chanting.

Instructions for the associated yoga pose:

Sit in a comfortable position with the elbows bent and tucked in. They'll need to be held against the ribcage tightly. This yoga is done with extended forearms outstretched to the front of the body with the palms facing upwards.

Sa Ta Na Ma

Pronunciation: Saa, Taa, Naa, Maa.

Meaning: This describes the eternal cycle of life.

Infinity; totality of the cosmos, including expansiveness and emotion. Life, from the beginning of birth to infinity, including strength and transformation. The death or transformation, and universal love. The rebirth and communication.

In the art of kundalini yoga, this mantra is used to increase an individual's intuition, and to balance the brain hemispheres, physically speaking. It's also chanted to create an individual's destiny. This mantra may also be used as a beginning point for healing and/or transformation.

What is Sun Gazing?

We receive vitamin D, solar energy, and warmth for power from many of our electronic utilities in the modern world. In fact, the sun is one of the most abundant sources of natural energy for life on Earth.

Within the Vedic system, there's a daily routine called *Sun Gazing* that students of any age can practice (using caution). According to Ayurveda practice, sun gazing has some very amazing benefits, and these aren't only for the physical health of individuals, but also for their spiritual development and mental health, too.

Benefits Can Include:

- More energy
- Increased production of the feel-good hormones (serotonin and melatonin)
- Improved eyesight
- Reduction of hunger pains because the body is nourished by the sunshine

- Growth and stimulation of the pineal gland
- Aiding the release of internal emotional blocks
- Increased personal potential

Please Note: This practice is only meant for practice during the first hour of sunrise, or the last hour before the sun is setting. UV rays can damage the eyesight, and so this cautionary measure is of the utmost importance.

Hira Ratan Manek Brought Sun Gazing to the Western World

It was Hira Ratan Manek who gave this practice its name and brought it to the Western world. He's more widely known as "HRM" and is the founder of the *Solar Healing Center*.

Hira Ratan Manek is famous for his ability to live off solar energy and water alone. His claims are quite incredible. At times, he claims to have buttermilk, tea, or coffee for social purposes only, but states in his own words that, "The sun can be used to heal the mind, body, and spirit." He also says that as a result of sun gazing, individuals can have better mental, emotional, physical, and spiritual health, overall.

Hira Ratan Manek has gone through 3, pivotal, long term fasts, and during these allocated times, he was under the strict supervision and observation of various medical and scientific teams. And this was done to provide statistical evidence of the benefits to this practice, as well as for his safety assurance.

Fasting by Hira Ratan Manek

Hira Ratan Manek's first fast went for 211 days in the years 1995 and 1996 in India. Dr. C.K. Ramachandran, a medical expert on Ayurvedic medicine, directed the study during that timeframe.

The second fast went for an unbelievable 411 days and began closely after the last one. During this time, Hira Ratan Manek had no food at all. The same study was also directed by an international team of 21 doctors and scientists, and this was led by Dr. Sudhir Shah and occurred in India.

The last (and third) fast went for 130 days, and this took place in the U.S. at *Thomas Jefferson University* and at the *University of Philadelphia*.

The Findings from Sun Gazing Studies by Vinny Pinto (using 56 participants)

1. Health improvements, especially among women.
2. People who practiced for more than 5 years and who gazed midday (instead of the hour after sunrise and hour before sunset) were more likely to report adverse or negative effects.
3. 35 out of the 51 participants reported "increased or greatly increased energy" while only 1 participant reported reduced energy.
4. The number of individuals who reported a "decreased need for solid food" was approximately equal to the number of individuals who reported "no significant change

in the need for food." Only one individual in the study reported an increased need for food.

5. Individuals who had sun gazed for at least 1 year and for at least 4 times per week were far more likely to report a decreased need for solid foods.
6. The most spoken about physical, spiritual, and mental experiences reported from sun gazing were those of joy, bliss, peace, and calmness.
7. No individuals from the study reported a decrease in their physical health, and all individuals reported that their health was either the same or had improved.

The HRM method is safe and popular:

If individuals are going to change this method in any way, they *must* do the research and not attempt to stare at the sun during the times where UV radiation is more present, or stare at the sun for longer than the recommended times.

> *A word of caution: You can change this method with how often you practice it, however, and for your intentions behind doing so, but you should try to adhere to the general guidelines so that you don't injure your eyesight or allow for permanent retinal damage, as this is very serious.*

The HRM Practice of Sun Gazing

Always stand barefoot on the bare earth. This helps the individual to keep grounded and can also enhance the benefits of sun gazing.

As you are staring at the sunshine, you should visualize the energy from the sun coming into your physical body and bringing your body and cells rejuvenating light.

Sun Gazing - Day 1

Start by spending a maximum of 10 seconds on the first day and do so by looking directly at the sun during the safe hours mentioned earlier. Continue this practice daily until you have reached the total of 44 minutes. This should take between 9 to 10 months and will be dependent upon the weather.

Sun Gazing - Day 2 to Day 10 & Onwards

On the second day, the individual should aim to do the practice for 20 seconds, and each day after that, add a further 10 seconds to the previous day. So, at the 10-day mark, the individual would be looking at the sun for a total of 100 seconds.

According to Hira Ratan Manek, this methodology is so that all individuals may gain the benefits described above from sun gazing. Everyone who practices sun gazing will generally report differently, as all individuals are not the same.

Important Note: This method also stipulates that the individual practicing sun gazing will need to walk for 45 minutes each day for the 6 days following the completion of their 9 to 10 months of sun gazing. After this stipulation by Hira Ratan Manek, the individual should make a conscious effort to walk barefoot upon the earth, preferably in the sunshine (whenever possible), or as time allows. During this time, the individual should remain centered and see what comes up (either mentally or spiritually speaking).

A Plethora of Information to Behold

This chapter has been full of a lot of information to take 'on board,' and so it would be wise to look over it again and even take notes, or perhaps highlight the most interesting parts.

The beauty of Ayurveda is that you can take what you need and give yourself each part of the information in 'bite-sized' elements, allowing you to learn and understand one part more fully before you move on to the next part or understanding.

A helpful 'rule of thumb' is to know your own dosha, and even the important people around you too, so that you can familiarize yourself with the characteristics and needs of each dosha. This information can help you gain benefits in all areas of Ayurvedic medicine, with relation to diet, meditation, yoga, chanting, earthing, and even sun gazing. The doshas are the main basis of Ayurveda, and so to understand these first and foremost is key, either as a student or as a future practitioner who helps others someday.

The most important part of Ayurveda is, in fact, all of it. It's the combination of all practices which allow the student to know and understand themselves within their own body, mind, and spiritual aspects, as well. The further you go with Ayurveda, the deeper can be the sense of connectedness that you have to it, in fact. And there's always something more to learn. And even through the practices, there can always be growth, too.

The most beautiful part of Ayurveda is all its parts, and that they can be flexible enough to suit the individual who practices them. There are multiple forms of dietary inclusions or exclusions, various meditation practices which suit doshas, chanting (or mantra) forms, earthing (or grounding) techniques, and other medicinal focuses to enable an individual to feel truly at home with this 5000-year-old way of medicine, a way which has also been backed by science and philosophy over the thousands of years of its existence, and in modern times, too.

The subsequent chapters will help the reader to practice Ayurveda techniques (which do not involve a practitioner), and this is so the student can incorporate the practices as well as the principles of Ayurvedic medicine, on the whole. In fact, learning how to utilize Ayurveda in everyday life, and fitting it into a busier, more modern schedule is key. Additionally, using the practices and principles can help the individual to feel better, even in a modern, busy world.

You might like to ask yourself, "When was the last time I studied or practiced something new to aid my health, my longevity, and my spiritual nature?" This question will give you insight before we begin on the next part of our understanding of Ayurveda. Let's 'dive in' now...

Chapter 7: Mindfulness as Both a Principle and a Practice

Why Is Practicing Mindfulness Important?

In truth, the mind is not a great fit for how and where we live. And yet, by practicing the art of mindfulness throughout your Ayurvedic journey, the individual can have the power to respond to their environment both differently and peacefully. Additionally, the mind can take us to all sorts of places via perception, but it's not always the right place, especially if it stays in the past or moves forward into the future in seemingly negative ways.

Human beings evolved over 200,000 years ago. The body and mind are the result of an incredible progression of adaptations brought about by a combination of random and genetic mutations, including inheritance, and reproductive factors.

We could say that these adaptations enabled the human race to survive some of the harshest environments on Earth. Including living in small, tight-knit groups, and tackling monumental challenges together. You might even say, and according to Cosmides and Tooby (2013), that humans were "on a camping trip that lasted a lifetime, and they had to solve many different kinds of problems well to survive and reproduce."

We know from history, that human nature excelled at focusing on short-term, local problems. We are exceptionally ingenious at finding food, seeking shelter, and avoiding being eaten by predators, but we're not very successful at tackling less immediate challenges like climate change, war, pandemics, obesity, and the plight of refugees, however.

But after 1000s of years of relative stability, the last few 100 generations (or so) have seen incredible cultural revolutions. These have occurred within farming, technology, and industry too, and have dramatically impacted the way we eat, sleep, communicate, and survive.

The biggest issue is that: the human mind has failed to keep up with our ever-changing lifestyles. And, generally, the brain, including all its processes, is no longer a good fit for the modern world. It's also true that evolutionary psychologists state this as being "psychological mismatches." The lack of alignment with the brain, therefore, impacts our ability to cope.

Many times, individuals become depressed, stressed, and anxious. But it doesn't have to be this way at all. And Ayurveda can connect individuals with a better way, in fact.

Saving a Nation's Health

In 2015, the *Mindful Nation Report* was published by the UK government. Its goals were different to any other policy document that been given prior. And using what is known as "positive psychology" to change an entire nation was thoroughly suggested.

The authors of this policy aimed to find a way to:

1. Improve mental health across the United Kingdom.
2. Increase creativity and productivity within the economy.
3. Help individuals who were suffering from long term health conditions.

One of the most exciting things the policy tried to do was to encourage "...the flourishing and wellbeing of a healthy nation." Interestingly, the report showed that up to 10% of the UK population (who were of adult age) were experiencing and living with depression, with only 1 in 3 individuals receiving support.

If we look at other countries, the statistics reflected are similar, with many individuals feeling overly stressed, anxious, obviously gaining weight, and becoming more and more unwell each and every year. Within traditional spirituality, like Ayurveda, it all stems from the mind as well as through behavioural choice and physical acts (like eating more, lack of exercise, overthinking, etc.)

Mindfulness Holds the Solution

Very interestingly too, the 2015 UK report found that the best way to tackle the problem was to encourage mindfulness as a practice within the workplace, and within education, healthcare, and the criminal justice system, too. This small (but simple) step was free, easy to do, and something which could be done almost anywhere, both safely and effectively.

Already, millions of people around the world practice the art of mindfulness. It's seen as a safe, natural, and as an easy-to-do approach for an individual's mental health, in fact. Imagine a world full of mindful people...

What is Mindfulness?

Being mindful means that the individual needs to pay attention to what's happening within the mind, the physical body, and within their immediate environment, as well. It's a case of being be present, while at the same time being compassionate and curious, too.

Mindfulness is not a complex task. Actually, it improves in response to a straightforward set of meditation practices which develops an increased awareness of sensations, thought patterns, and feelings, overall. And combined with increased passion and kindness, mindfulness improves the individual's capacity to cope by way of identifying the options available at any given point in time.

Overall, mindfulness can lead to a greater, healthier wellbeing, including aiding mental clarity, and even the increased ability to care for the self and others. The practice of mindfulness can be as simple as an awareness of the breath and the physical body at any given moment. Individuals can observe their thoughts and emotions as they come and go, before gently returning the prime focus to the body's physical sensations, whilst remaining compassionate, curious, and accepting. It's kind of like admiring the body from a distance of sorts and then realizing that the feelings and sensations can be treated immediately; with a new breath and/or a new thought which is positive and calming.

The Benefits of Mindfulness

Over the last decade, countless research studies have proven that mindfulness has many significant cognitive, psychological, and physical benefits to individuals.

The benefits of mindfulness are sometimes stated on multiple platforms of the media, where the data continues to expose benefits in many facets of a person's life. The practices are quite simple but not always easy to incorporate into each day, especially if the individual has a negative mindset, or is unwilling to practice mindfulness regularly. Let's take a look at some of the fundamental benefits of mindfulness now.

The Psychological Benefits of Mindfulness

Increased happiness, increased compassion, increased life satisfaction, increased relationship satisfaction, increased work satisfaction, increased sense of meaning, decreased stress, decreased depression, and decreased anxiety.

The Cognitive Benefits of Mindfulness

Increased attention, increased memory, increased creativity, increased innovation, reduced mind wandering, increased problem solving, and increased test scores.

The Physical Benefits of Mindfulness

Improved immune function, reduced hypertension, decreased chronic pain, improved cardiovascular function, decreased levels of cortisol, better sleep quality, cortical thickening, and improved neural integration.

Great Tips for Achieving Mindfulness Daily

Stop What You're Doing and Take a Breath

Take a moment to feel the sensation of your breath. Create an intentional space for resettling yourself, doing so even with just that first breath, and this will help to keep you calmer and more focused throughout your day.

Put Down Your Phone

Your body's system is pulled toward the most stimulating thing around you, and your phone was designed to be exactly that. Holding onto a phone may temporarily help with boredom or feel like freedom, but it also allows you to tune out many important sensations, including your surroundings. Make time each day to put your phone out of reach and take note of the difference. You'll feel more present, too.

Do One Task at a Time

Sometimes, we can try to prioritize tasks by handling them as they come in, even if it means starting a new task while various others are already being dealt with. A huge component of mindfulness is doing only one thing at a time: a practice of giving all your attention and awareness to the task at hand. It will also allow the brain to cope far better, too.

Find Mindful Moments in Daily Tasks

Mindfulness involves the practice of intentionally doing one thing at a time and becoming more aware of the task *and* your response to doing it. The next time you're doing the dishes, folding laundry, or any other remedial task, make it mindful. Notice your physical sensations. Is it possible to allow yourself to get immersed into the experience so that it becomes enjoyable?

Notice What You Already Do

There are various ways to practice mindfulness with movement, and you can make it as active (or non-active) as you like If you already dance or exercise in some way that helps you to feel more centered and present in the current moment, then that could be your mindfulness practice. Or perhaps your practice might be as simple as paying attention to the feeling of your feet on the ground as you walk. It's not about what you focus your attention on really, but that you take the time to consistently practice holding your awareness on just one thing, always taking note of what comes up.

Ideas to Build Yourself Through Mindfulness within the Community

1. You could build a community with others also integrating mindfulness skills.
2. You might like to learn multiple practices for ongoing self-care and wellness.
3. You might study and understand more fully the science behind these practices.
4. You could use specific tools for mindfully managing all aspects of your life.

The Realization of Our Lives Before Mindfulness is Key

The individual's mind is consistently filled with 'chatter,' and the overall view of the world might even become tainted and distorted, including the ability to be present, or (as the opposite) becoming lost. This can happen because life is often frantic and can get thoroughly exhausting. And this will impact the individual's happiness, education, health, work, and even the economy, if we look at the bigger scale and join communities together.

The Best Plan Towards Mindfulness

There's growing proof that mindfulness-based therapies offer thorough support for mental health. Ayurveda promotes this within its practices as a necessity. Perhaps less well known, these techniques can dramatically improve physical wellbeing, psychological wellbeing, and cognitive wellbeing, too. We looked at this a little earlier within this chapter.

Mindfulness takes the individual beyond coping and merely making do with their current lifestyle. The techniques help people to see the world differently, and to grow and flourish, and even live a more compassionate, fuller, and more fulfilled life.

If mindfulness were something available in stores for purchase, it would be "out of stock" on a regular basis. Teaching nations how to do this would benefit the whole of humanity, in fact. The whole planet would be less stressed, calmer, feel less worry, and feel better, overall.

Stress & Mindfulness

In recent studies, researchers found that undergraduates higher in mindfulness were less stressed, both physiologically and psychologically. Studies were also conducted during traumatic climate events, like during severe thunderstorms, hurricanes, and more. According to science, it seems that mindfulness helps individuals manage existing stress and that mindfulness also offers protection from future upset, even if it's dramatic.

Happiness & Mindfulness

Some scientific studies have confirmed how important mindfulness is in managing our perception of happiness. Where happiness is not just something that feels good, but something which might offer protection against disease and even death, or at least the fear of it. It's also true, that maintaining a positive mindset is crucial to keeping healthy.

When mindfulness training was given to patients (in 2020) with the disease known as diabetes, not only did their measures of happiness increase, but as well, their blood glucose levels were better controlled. Similar improvements were shown in people with low mood, anxiety, and even clinical depression.

Memory & Mindfulness

Mindfulness has been scientifically proven to have a positive effect on stress, as well as a benefit to getting better sleep and helping with memory. As a result, significantly upping our mindfulness improves our chances of recalling information. And this is great news.

Just a 3-minute session provides immediate improvements to memory performance, according to science. It's so effective that the studies suggest that a brief mindfulness session could even reduce false recall for eyewitness statements in a court session.

Creativity & Mindfulness

Recently, research has also discovered that mindfulness sessions aid focus and increase creativity in both individuals and group settings.

Other cognitive benefits have been seen, too. Mindfulness fundamentally improves the individual's ability to tackle problems. It reduces the wandering of the mind and offers the increased capacity (as a potential) in the rest of the brain for extra cognitive processing to occur.

Genetics & Mindfulness

Not only do we see improvements in the individual's general health, but research has deemed that mindfulness improves telomerase activity within the physical being. In fact, the vital enzyme controls cellular aging, and the age-related decline of the entire body. So, longevity is the possible outcome here. This really does put the "wow" factor on mindfulness as a key 'ingredient' within the practice of Ayurveda.

Immune Function & Mindfulness

Immunity is a crucial factor in the maintenance of good health, particularly for anyone with a compromised immune function. A study (in 2019) revealed that women in early stages of breast cancer who received mindfulness training, not only reduced their fatigue, stress, and sleep disturbances, but also optimized their immune systems, too.

Can the Practice of Mindfulness Change Your Brain?

Your brain is not completely fixed, in fact, it has elasticity, so you *can* change it. Grow to who *you* want to be! There's that famous saying, "You can do anything that you put your mind to." And this should have been written about mindfulness, although it probably was.

Scientists used to believe, that after a certain age, the human brain stopped changing. But in recent years, research has proved this to be a false claim. So, no matter what age the individual is, they will never stop being able to change their mind, quite literally so.

Generally, genetics and our early years partly define who we are, but the rest is completely malleable. This realization is hugely important and freeing. We can understand that our parents and our upbringing matters, but the rest of who we are is truly a choice we make. We can either see this as a crisis, the seeming terror that we must take responsibility for who we are, or we can see it as an opportunity to be who, or what, we want to be within our own lives.

The scientific discovery of neuroplasticity means that the human brain continually develops throughout its life. And so, at any age, you can change your brain's physical way of working, and Ayurvedic techniques can help with this. Additionally, it makes sense in evolutionary terms, that humans utilize essential pathways, and shift those which serve no purpose.

Why do humans remain with their old patterns of thinking and behavior?

This is mostly because it requires effort to practice. There are no free passes. The question truly becomes, *what do you want to grow?* And here is where mindfulness comes in.

Mindfulness & the Brain

We've already seen the positive impacts of mindfulness on the workings of the brain. These are the psychological and cognitive processing which occurs. And, we also have clear evidence that mindfulness affects, not only the 'software' of the brain, but also the 'hardware' too.

A study (in 2018) of peer-reviewed research using functional magnetic resonance imaging (fMRI), showed that mindfulness changed activity in the brain's insular cortex. This is the part of the brain that's involved in an unbelievable variety of functioning, including decision making processes, sensory processing, and the handling of an individual's feelings and emotions. This part of the brain is also associated with the awareness of internal reactions, which might more commonly be understood as the individual's ability to be present in the moment.

Other scientific studies show that mindfulness increases the production of brain-derived neurotrophic factor (or BDNF). This is an essential protein which helps to encourage the survival, development, and the plasticity of neurons within the brain.

Here, every piece of data presented as scientific evidence points to the ability of mindfulness to be able to rewire the brain, impacting the individual's learning abilities, memory recall, and overall cognition.

Mindfulness in Schools

Institutions around the world are beginning to see the myriad of potentiality of mindfulness within the realm of education.

The benefits include:
- Improving academic results
- Increasing children's mental health
- Aiding character building
- Aiding resilience and coping mechanisms

As a result, many schools around the world have focused on resources by way of strengthening these key elements and in helping to promote overall wellbeing, naturally. And Ayurveda has been trying to do this for around 5,000 years. Just imagine that mindfulness was implicated into schooling and education from its earliest beginnings. The world (as we know it) might be a different place right now.

Scientific evidence concludes that mindfulness improves the capacity of a child's brain to manage cognitive processes, like problem solving, reasoning, and memory. In the long run, this ability to understand and manage emotions predicts an individual's ability to maintain their health, their income, and the likelihood of criminal behavior in later life.

Mindfulness is a Big Part of the Answer in the Workplace

Much research is still in its beginning stages, but multiple world-leading companies seem to realize it's got a big part to play within the workplace.

Some businesses have found considerable success with employee programs which promote mindfulness. Not only has it seen significant productivity improvements, but it's also recognized as the reason many of these employers are ranked as being the best in the world. Their staff can feel the differences.

Research shows improvements to mental wellbeing across a wide variety of professions, as well. Including teachers, policemen (and women), and firefighters, too. It's also led to some unexpected improvements where mindfulness may also reduce racial and age-related discrimination. This is a huge plus in the division of many individuals within the workplace.

All in all, the workplace can be more productive, happier, more positive, and fairer for employees, overall. The major downside, however, is that mindfulness can't correct excessive workloads, poor management skills, and a bad or negative working environment. Mindfulness does have the ability to build more productive and compassionate staff, and individuals who are focused on their tasks with greater clarity, though.

Mindfulness is for Everyone

Mindfulness changes a person in 3 poignant ways: psychologically, cognitively, and physically. As the individual chooses mindfulness, they're actively deciding to be happier, less stressed, more creative, and more focused. The improvements in sleep quality, immunity, and life expectancy are scientifically and evidence based, too.

The most attractive part of mindfulness is that it also offers an unbelievable opportunity to enjoy and grow in life. Individuals can learn how to stop, take time out, breathe, focus, admire beauty, and live from a place of compassion and joy.

Chapter 8: Ayurveda as an Advanced Practice in the Modern Busy World

Why is the ancient wisdom of Ayurveda so relevant today for our busy, modern-day lives?

Ayurveda is a simple and practical holistic healing system with principles that come from ancient Vedas of India. We are already familiar that it's one of the oldest forms of health science in the known world.

Ayurveda's aim is to understand the individual's personal constitution (Prakruti) and its relationship to the laws of nature in reaching a perfect and harmonious balance within the body, the soul, and the mind. Understanding the individual's constitution plays a key role in how effectively someone can live out their own life. Ayurveda is a preventing and relieving medicine of the body and mind through self-observation and self-care.

Self-Care in a Busy World

Self-care is described as any internal action the individual takes to care for their own physical health, as well as their mental and emotional wellbeing. Terms used to describe this concept are self-soothing, purposeful, regular, deliberate, and self-initiated.

Self-care is often an area most individuals will overlook. Being selfless is an admirable trait, and those with bigger responsibilities demonstrate this daily, but doing self-care is much more imperative so that they have enough energy to offer those relationships and show up as the best version of themselves.

In fact, the better care we take of our physical body and our mental and emotional wellbeing, the more balanced we are. Self-care, therefore, leads the individual to becoming self-aware.

The Most Ancient Wisdom Knew This

The ancient wisdom of Ayurveda utilizes and shows individuals various ways to maintain balance within as the variables of everyday life change. Seasons change, work might change, localities of residence might change, relationships change, and we get older. The only constant in life is change. If individuals adjust accordingly (internally) to stresses or external factors, they can remain in a state of relative equilibrium and good health, too.

Having a daily routine invites health in and brings vitality and a sense of clarity into the day. Having an appropriate routine or healthful habits is one of the most grounding and nurturing things you could do for yourself. Some examples might be rising with the sun, starting the day with a warm drink of ginger, lemon and honey to flush the system and awaken digestion, scraping the tongue to remove toxins, and morning movement like yoga and meditation. Yoga and meditation can aid in toileting and allow the mind to become focused for the day ahead. Self-massage with oil is wonderful, too, and is extremely effective in keeping individuals both balanced and grounded.

Eating Well & Herbs & Spices with Healing Power

Ayurveda admires the healing power of spices and herbs and what's best to eat for an individual, including how, when and the amounts, too It gives specific therapeutic treatments (via professional practitioners) to improve and eliminate illnesses of the body and mind. Ayurveda looks for the root cause of an illness rather than just treating its symptoms.

We live in a world full of electricity, technology, family pressures, financial burdens, stresses, social expectations, and unhealthy processed foods. This is far from the type of lives the Indian sages and scholars led. They enjoyed revered lives of self-inquiry, joining with nature, living by way of nature's rhythms, and a spiritual placement of true intention. And by studying the ways in which they lived their lives with mindfulness and intention, individuals can find this state of balance amidst the chaos of their busy, stressful and modern lives.

Becoming More Mainstream

"Ayurvedic medicine is ancient, its resurgence is necessary because we do need the proper balance in our medical approach." - *Maya Tiwari*

Ayurvedic Usage

If we look at turmeric, for example, this an excellent root in Ayurvedic formulations and meals, known for its active ingredient curcumin and its anti-inflammatory and antibacterial properties. It's now so prevalent on the market and very accepted, too.

In some cases, pharmaceutical drugs have failed, and so the principles of Ayurveda and its herbs have made headway, succeeding with great efficacy, in fact. And even more powerful is the integration of modern medicine with the use of ancient Ayurvedic principles to reach new levels of healing, getting results for some patients where every other treatment or drug might have failed. Seeking out an experienced Ayurvedic practitioner is key.

Ayurveda is great for everyone. And as individuals rush through their overly demanding lives, it's important to take some time out to slow down, nurture, live with harmony with nature, and nourish the individual by utilizing the laws of ancient Ayurveda.

True Health Promotion

Ayurvedic theory and principles focus upon the individual, not on group or community health as might be the case within Western medicine principles.

Interestingly too, there's no public health branch for Ayurveda. Ayurvedic theory has a tradition to improving the health status for the individual, and by way of their uniqueness. Health promotion concepts, on the other hand, may be enriched by an understanding of the tridosha theory too, mixed with ecological health concepts, yoga, and nutrition with other concepts from Ayurveda.

For individuals, finding out their dosha is key, and if there are ailments, diseases, or conditions, then seeing a practitioner of Ayurveda is the first main step towards health and longevity. Many practitioners will be aware of Western medicine principles if both are to be utilized.

Loving the Art of Yoga

Sometimes, the most prescribed form of health care by practitioners (of Ayurveda) is yoga. In India, many traditional Vaidas teach yoga as an integral part of their practice. Yoga, remember, is the Sanskrit word which comes from "yug," meaning "to join or to unite." And in its most basic understanding, yoga therefore means "union," and in the spiritual sense it pertains to joining the individual soul with the universal spirit, and then moving to join the mind, body, and soul together.

Swami Yogananda said, "The consciousness of a perfected yogi is effortlessly identified not with a narrow body but with the universal structure." And so, it's clear that yoga is a holistic science which embraces many aspects: the physical, the moral, the social, the mental, and the spiritual wellbeing of the individual. It does its efficacy with wholeness and with the acceptance of the individual.

Many branches of yoga are really just meditations in various forms. We could say, that yogic practice is partly an attempt to cultivate the individual's powers of adaptation and adjustment via an internal transitioning, so as to withstand all of the external changes such as disease-causing agents and other changes in the outside world.

Encouragement of the 3 steps should be the goal for individuals practicing yoga:

1. The cultivation of correct psychological attitudes
2. The reconditioning of the neuro-muscular and neuro-glandular systems and the entire body to allow the individual to withstand greater stress and strain, all at the same time.
3. To begin emphasizing a healthful diet, and the encouragement of the natural processes of elimination, whenever necessary, by way of detoxes and baths. This might be recommended by an Ayurvedic practitioner.

Many traditionalists believe that the goals of Ayurveda and yoga are the same: to allow people to attain self-realization. The major difference being that yoga trains people to attain mental and physical strength without the help of external needs.

Additionally, Ayurvedic theory and principles assume that some individuals aren't able to be disciplined enough to develop this kind of strength on their own, and so practitioners of Ayurveda provide various remedies and medicines for this purpose, as well as for the express treatment of disease.

The Importance of Treating Disease

In general, in Ayurveda, there are 2 types of medicines:

1. Those that promote resistance of the body and promote vitality.
2. Those which cure disease.

In Ayurveda, preventive measures allow a broad variety of regimes and will be given by the practitioner to the client:

1. Swastavritta is personal hygiene. Here dinacaya (a daily routine) incorporates tooth brushing, using mouth wash, tongue scraping, bathing, exercising, eating, and sleeping, etc.
2. Ritucarya are the regimes of diet which are to be followed during the different seasons of the year.
3. Sadvritta is the social behavior and conduct of the individual based upon religious rituals and practices.
4. Rasayana and vajeekarana are utilizing, rejuvenating, and virilizing agents to prevent aging, to give longevity, to promote immunity against disease, and to assist in improving the individual's mental focus.

The second aim of Ayurveda is to give respite to suffering patients with the attempt to cure disease. Here, there are 8 main branches of Ayurveda (astanga sanigraha):

1. Kaaya chikithasa – for general medicine which includes internal purification and curative treatment.
2. Baala chikithasa – for children's health.
3. Shalya chikithsa – for surgery.
4. Oordhwaanga chikithasa – for the eyes, ears, nose, and throat.
5. Graha chikithsa – for mental health.
6. Damshtraa chikithsa – for toxicology.
7. Jaraa chikithsa – for elderly care focused upon prolonging life, arousing memory, and strengthening vital organs against disease and decay.

8. Vrushaa chikithsa – for the science of aphrodisiacs/virility/ rejuvenation, and for increasing the pleasures of sexuality to make individuals more intimate with partners. It also assists in improving fertility, including treatments for faulty sperm and reproductive fluids.

The Ayurvedic forms of treatment are purposefully plant derived, with some use of mineral based substances as well. Ayurvedic remedies from practitioners are generally not made from any animal sources. These anciently derived remedies make use of the powers of nature to restore human beings to a more natural state of balance.

Additionally, herbs and minerals are used singularly (or in the form of compounds) which are professionally made. Ayurvedic pharma utilizes the use of pastes, juice powders, cold infusions, infusion, decoctions, decoctions in milk, extracts, pills, medicated spirited liquids, medicated clarified butter, and many more.

The practitioner will use 4 healing factors, which include:

Samshamanan – The pacification of the deranged or agitated body which gives rise to disease.

Samshodhanam – The cleansing. Done internally, where purgatives or enemas are used, or externally, where surgery, plasters or cauterization of affected parts are utilized.

Sadvritt: The understanding – The conduct, where mentality, bodily acts, and speech are viewed and assessed.

Pathyahara: The diet, using food as medicine, including herbs and compounds.

Punchamahabhutas The Ayurvedic Five Element Theory.

The 5 Element Theory where ether, air, fire, water and earth, or the punchamahabhutas, are the foundation of all existence. They're present in all animate and inanimate entities. And here, energy and matter are considered as being interchangeable.

Although the elements and how they combine are different, the Chinese Five Element Theory parallels this too, in that everything on earth is said to be dominated by one of these elements and their constant interplay with the universe. This combined with those of yin and yang, explain all change and activity within the realm of nature.

Ether - Non-resistance, sound, and essence

Air - Expansion, sound, and touch

Fire - Heat, luminosity, sound, color, and touch

Water - Liquidity, sound, taste, touch, color, and touch

Earth - Roughness, sound, touch, color, taste, and smell

The human body, the food, all plants, all animals, and all minerals contain the bhutas. From the bhutas, the dhatus (or constructing elements) are made or formed. They are responsible for form and function within the organism.

The Dhatus

Rasa – The equivalent to plasma. It contains nutrients from digested food and nourishes all the tissues, organs, and the systems, too.

Rakta – The equivalent to blood. It governs oxygen in all the tissues and vital organs to maintain life.

Mamsa – The equivalent to flesh/muscle. It covers the delicacy of the vital organs, performs the movements of the joints, and maintains the physical strength of the physical body.

Meda – The equivalent to fat. It maintains the lubrication and moisture of all the tissues.

Asthma – The equivalent to bone. It gives support to the body's structure.

Majja – The equivalent to marrow and nerves. It fills up the space within bones and carries the motor and sensory impulses throughout the body.

Shukra & Artava – The equivalent to sperm and the reproductive fluid/tissues. They contain the ingredients of all tissues and are responsible for procreation (making life).

Disorders in the Balance of the Physical Body

Disorders within the balance of an individual's physical body will directly affect the dhatus. Health may be gained through proper nutrition, ongoing bodily care, movement through exercise (note that excessive sweating and rapid pulse and respiratory rates are not recommended in Ayurveda), and via rejuvenation. Disturbed dhatus are directly involved with the disease process.

The Macrocosm & the Microcosm

According to holistic principles, the smallest particle of the universe is the universe in its smallest form. The interaction between the universe and the individual takes place through the course of intake and output matter. Here, the universe is said to be the macrocosm and other matter, including human beings, are said to be the microcosm. The punchamahabhuta principles are connected here. These holistic principles state that there's a unity and oneness in the universe and that all is connected.

The Punchamahabhuta

We might it explain the 'sameness' (or samanya) of 'self' (or purusha) and 'nature' (or prakruti) as the underlying principle of all Ayurvedic practices. The profound and ecological principle, which embodies the understanding that the individual's body, mind, and soul is connected to all other life forms in the universe. In Ayurveda, this principle is seen throughout different forms which govern the modalities of health promotion, disease prevention, and curative care for all age groups.

Nutrition is a Definitive Key Element

As well as yoga, meditation, and having a daily routine, the nourishment of the physical body is central to Ayurvedic health promotion concepts. No distinction is made between that of food and medicine, so the kitchen becomes the pharmacy, and cooking and pharmacology are considered one.

Interestingly, all food is considered to have some type of medicinal value, too. A healthful diet is considered preventive of disease and can, therefore, substitute for stronger medicine. Here, by changing dietary habits, the individual may be cured without using any medicine, and in contrast, with a myriad of good medicines (foods and herbs), diseases of the individual can't be cured if the food is wrong. And so, the right food is the key to good health, overall.

It makes sense, that the selection and preparation of fresh, organic, and chemical-free food is the key player for the cultivation of vibrant health, and for the treatment of disease.

Foods that Harm & Foods That Heal

Beneficial food, including herbs and condiments promote body growth and injurious food produces disease. Here, the food is of 3 types: svastha vrittikara (or life giving), vyadhi prashaman (or therapeutic), and dosha prashamanam (used as a pacifier for imbalanced doshas).

Now we can remember the different tastes: sweet, sour, astringent, salty, pungent, and bitter. Each dosha is enhanced and can be unbalanced by the intake of certain tastes. Complex nutritional theory within the Ayurveda realm utilizes several applications of taste for diet and medicinal preparations.

The individual's daily intake should contain all 6 tastes in significant proportions.

An Insight on Sweet Foods

Sweet foods are for body building and energy production; they're found in carbohydrates, fats, and albumen.

An Insight on Bitter & Sour & Salty Foods

A percentage of bitter and sour components in food promotes the secretion of the gastric juices and sharpens the appetite. Many acid substances aid digestion. They contain vitamins, in fact. And vitamin C (for example) works well, and also salts (from healthful foods, not processed foods) form the basis of minerals needed to maintain the body's electrolytic balance.

An Insight on Astringent Foods

Astringents are foods containing tannin. They stop over-activity in the small intestine and ensure that the food is digested for longer and more thoroughly, too.

Each dosha has specific dietary recommendations. If individuals eat foods which are not recommended for their particular dosha-type, the Ayurvedic philosophy is quite forgiving, and it's definitely possible to counter the negative effects of those foods. An example is: people of the vata dosha ought to be careful about consuming foods which produce too much wind, as vata may be imbalanced by over-consumption of beans, cabbage, or cauliflower, especially if they haven't been soaked before cooking, and so on. And so, to counter this, gently chewing on a raw clove, cardamom pods, or fennel seeds, will enable the juice to slowly pass through the digestive tract, and so vata individuals may alleviate some of the stress which was pushed into their system.

The 12 Food Groups of Ayurveda

In Ayurveda, there are 12 food groups which consist of: legumes, nuts, cereals, flesh, vegetables growing underneath the ground, fruits, sugar, wine, water, milk, fats and oils, and spices.

Ayurveda also has 4 categories of prepared food, which should be added into the daily diet of people of all doshas, unless they have allergies to them:

1. *Foods of normal consistency* like rice and bread, as examples.
2. *Liquids*, like milk, soup, and natural fruit juice, as examples.
3. *Tasteful foods* like chutneys, sweet and sour sauces, preserves, ketchups, and pastes, as examples.
4. *Crisp and chewy foods*, like nuts or salads, as examples.

Regulation of Digestion

An individual's intake and digestion are optimally regulated by the agni (or fire) of the physical body. The digestive system is like a flame which must be strong and able to burn fuel rapidly. Here, tiny flames must be given the purest and finest fuel very slowly, otherwise the flame will flicker and falter. Strong flames may be built up through proper nutrition and may create a stronger 'set of flames' which is able to withstand 'wetness' (or difficult to digest foods) with only a patch of smokiness. The goal of healthful eating is to enable true digestive vitality.

The Goal is Digestive Strength at Optimum Levels

The result of an individual having digestive strength is complete dietary freedom. To have complete freedom to live as the individual pleases, but also being aware enough to realize that physical health depends upon the strength of the digestive system. Therefore, the individual should be motivated enough to want to guard this precious resource of knowledge.

Listening to the Body, Intuitively

Eating well encourages true sensitivity, and 'hearing' the physical body's messages is key. Don't eat unless you feel hungry, and don't drink unless you feel thirsty. And so, listening to the body means that the individual is crystal clear about which food has beneficial and non-beneficial effects, because the stomach is being acknowledged more fully as the person feels their way.

Some important principles to help with intuitive eating:

1. Food should be hot (usually cooked).
2. Food should be tasty and easy to digest.
3. Food should be eaten in the proper amounts, not too much or too little. Here, 2 handfuls are recommended, so that the stomach is filled a third with food, a third with water, and a third with air.
4. Food should be eaten on an empty stomach, and after the last meal has been digested properly.
5. Foods should work together and not contradict one another in their actioning.
6. Foods should be eaten in pleasant surroundings with the proper equipment for their enjoyment.

7.   Eating shouldn't ever be rushed.
8.   Eating shouldn't be an overly long process.
9.   The individual should focus on the food while eating.
10. Only eating food that's relevant to the individual's particular dosha is necessary.

Seasonal Eating is Beneficial

Eating with the seasons assists the body in adjusting to the seasonal variations which change throughout the year. In each season, one or more doshas predominate. In wintertime, kapha gains strength, which promotes the growth and maintenance of the body's tissues, aids in strengthening immunity, and lubricates the joints, too. Kapha brings an abundance of mucus, which may lead to coughs, colds, and influenza, especially for children. The digestive power and appetite are more powerful during the long nights, so it's possible for individuals to cope with heavier foods and more of an abundance of them. It's the time for warm cooked grains, like oats, rice, soups, and heavier protein foods like beans, warm teas, honey, and heated milk. Be aware of allergies, though.

During the springtime, the doshas of vata and pitta thrive, with new beginnings being at the forefront, and the accumulated kapha and extra body weight being released by the individual's more active levels, because of avoiding the need for over-sleeping, and by choosing lighter, bitter, and fresher foods. A well-made 'tonic' of dark leafy greens can help in detoxifying the physical body, through the kidneys and the liver. Heavy, oily, sweet, and sour foods should be avoided, however.

The summer is dominated by pitta, and heat and dryness. The digestive fire, known as agni is exceptionally strong at this time and ought not be overworked with pitta foods of the spicier, hotter, more pungent, sour, oily, and saltier choices. Instead, moister, cooler, and liquid-type foods can satiate the pitta, like milk, seasonal fruits, rice, tofu, and aloe vera juice, as examples. Eating and drinking lightly is the aim to thriving in pitta climates, which promote a lot of perspiration, the decaying of food, and tissue loss.

In the fall (or springtime), vata is beginning to rise. The essence of vata is the pelvis (at the root and sacral chakras) which has implications of energy for both survival and security. Vata imbalances (like dry skin or aching joints) may become more apparent at this time. Warmer, moister, and more well-lubricated foods are necessary, with a focus on sweeter, sour, and saltier (foods which are naturally salty, not processed foods or adding salt to meals) tastes.

During the change of season, it's best to follow guidelines for the approaching season one week beforehand, and this is so the physical body has some adjustment time. Fasting is recommended too, for those who can do this without becoming unwell. And this occurs particularly for the kapha and pitta doshas to allow agni to burn away any build-up of toxins from the intestines, and to purify the whole system. It's also true that the stomach and intestines are treated with the utmost care, as it's difficult for the rest of the body to be diseased when they are looked after nutritionally. Interestingly too, most diseases are linked to disharmonious eating habits and/or eating foods which antagonize the physical body. Some holistic practitioners state that digestive disorders are the most common health problems seen and dealt with in modern times.

The Tridosha Theory

Ayurvedic theory is based upon the notion that observing nature is the best way to learn about the human physical body. From the 5 bhutas, which are found in the human body, comes the tridoshas.

A More In-Depth Look at the Doshas

From ether and air, the vata dosha is created.

From fire and water, the pitta dosha is created.

From water and earth, the kapha dosha is created.

Doshas are generally understood as the resting states, from which the mind/body constitutional types are created. They're powerful energy forces or inner principles within the human body which govern the entire being.

Ayurvedic theory understands that all human bodies are *not* equal, so there are 7 basic doshic prakrutis, or constitutions, stemming from vata, pitta and kapha, and their combinations known as: vata, pitta, kapha, vata-pitta, vata-kapha, pitta-kapha, and vata-pitta-kapha. An individual can, therefore, be uni-doshic, bi-doshic, or tri-doshic (where tri-doshic is a fully balanced individual, which is very rare).

So, vata, comes from the Sanskrit basis of "va" which means "motion," and "ganthana" which means "sensation." And so, vata begins all movement in the physical body and governs mainly all the nervous functions.

Pitta comes from the Sanskrit root of "tap," which means "heat." And so, pitta governs mostly the enzymes and hormones, respiration for digestion, the pigmentation, an individual's body temperature, the thirst, the eyesight, an individual's courage, and any secretions and excretions which are either the needs or the wastes of tissue combustion.

Kapha is from the Sanskrit root of "kena jelana phalatiiti" which means the "fruit" or "product of water." And so, kapha regulates the other two doshas and is the overseer for the connection of the joints, the solidness of the body and its substances, the individual's sexual power, and the person's strength and patience.

Knowing the Individual's Dosha Type is Paramount

Ayurvedic healthcare is worked out based upon determining the dosha of each individual, because, from the dosha, comes a general guide to the most appropriate dietary patterns, activity levels, and treatment options when dealing with imbalances which might cause disease.

Let's revisit some knowledge to revise or learning now.

Revisiting the 3 Ayurveda Principles

1. Vata is the energy of movement.
2. Pitta is the energy of digestion or metabolism.
3. Kapha is the energy of lubrication and structure.

Every individual has the qualities of vata, pitta, and kapha, but one is usually primary, one secondary, and the third is usually least dominant of all. The cause of disease in Ayurveda is viewed as a lack of proper cellular function, due to either the excess or deficiency of vata, pitta, or kapha.

Disease can also be attributed by the presence of toxins within the body, and this is important and a key understanding here. Many individuals don't realize the toxicity within their own bodies. And toxins can be present within the foods, medications, in allergens (like pet fur), in water sources, within the air, within the atmosphere, in fabrics or paints, and in chemicals or sprays found within a home, business, region, or locality.

This reminder is key, especially where human beings get caught eating and drinking foods which don't help them. Alcohol is one example and processed or 'dead' foods are another. The importance of keeping the body clean and pure is essential. The use of illicit and overly prescribed drugs is also linked to problems.

Remember too, that the body, the mind, and the consciousness all come together to maintain the right balance. They are easily and effectively viewed as different facets of an individual's beingness that makes up the whole person.

Looking at the 5 Great Elements

Remember, to learn how to balance the body, the mind, and the consciousness, this requires an understanding of how vata, pitta, and kapha work, and that they do so in combination with each other. As we already know, these are: space, air, fire, water, and earth.

The principles of vata, pitta, and kapha are combinations and extensions of these 5 elements which are brought about as patterns that are said to be present in all of creation. In the physical body, vata is the subtle energy of movement, pitta is the energy of digestion and metabolism, and kapha is the energy that forms the body's structure and its lubrication.

The Importance of Vata: The Subtle Energy Concerning Movement

This principle is composed of the elements *space* and *air*. As we know, it takes care of breathing, blinking, muscle and tissue movement, the pulsation of the heart, and every set of movements within the cytoplasm of the cells, including the cell membranes. When in order (or balance), vata allows creativity and flexibility. In disorder (or imbalance) vata allows fear and anxiety to take hold.

The Importance of Pitta: The Expression of the Body's Metabolic System

This principle is composed of the elements *fire* and *water*. As we know, it takes care of digestion, absorption, assimilation, nutrition, metabolism, physical body temperature. When in order (or balance), pitta allows understanding and intelligence. Out of order (or imbalance), pitta allows anger, hatred, narcissism, and jealousy.

The Importance of Kapha: The Thorough Energy Which Forms the Body's Structure

This principle is composed of the elements *earth* and *water*. As we know, it takes care of the bones, muscles, and the tendons. It holds everything together. In fact, kapha supplies the water for all body parts and systems. It proceeds to lubricate the joints, moisturize the skin, and maintain overall immunity within the physical body. When in order (or balance), kapha allows love, calmness, peace, and forgiveness. Out of order (or imbalance), it allows attachment, greed, and envy.

It's All About Balance...

To maintain balance and to promote health, it's thoroughly important to pay attention to all decisions related to an individual's wellbeing. Diet and lifestyle factors, which are appropriate to an individual's dosha type will strengthen the body, mind, and the consciousness, too.

The Complementary System of Healing

Remember, the basic difference between Ayurveda and Western medicine is important to understand. Western medicine generally focuses upon symptomatology and disease, and mostly uses drugs and surgery to rid the body of pathogens or diseased tissue.

The science used is for multiple individuals, as opposed to a unique look at the individual in question. It's true that many lives have been saved by this fixing approach. And, as we know, in some instances, surgery is encouraged by Ayurveda. However, drug reliance, because of the toxicity involved, often weakens the body. And Ayurveda's goal is strengthening, not weakening.

Ayurveda *does not* focus on the existence of disease. In fact, Ayurveda maintains that all life must be supported by energy which is in balance or "order." When there's minimal stress and the flow of energy within a person is balanced not disordered, and the body's natural defence systems will be strong enough to defend against disease.

Ayurveda is not a substitute for Western medicine. Always seek a practitioner's advice and do your own research with regards to your choices. Ayurveda can be used in conjunction with Western medicine, however. It's up to the individual how they take care of their own health, however.

We all have times when we don't feel quite right, and we might even recognize that we're out of balance. Sometimes, we might have seen a practitioner only to be told that there's nothing truly wrong at all.

According to Ayurvedic philosophy, what's really occurring is that this imbalance has not yet become recognizable as a full-blown illness or disease. It is, however, serious enough to make the person notice some level of discomfort. So, if you're keen to practice Ayurveda, the medicinal part should always be done by a true, professional practitioner.

Some Things to Ask Know Before Seeing an Ayurvedic Practitioner

If you've never worked with an Ayurvedic practitioner before, you might find the diagnostic and treatment procedures a bit confusing. To make the whole process easier for you, here are some valuable questions to ask. During your initial consultation, asking questions to help you understand how

Ayurveda works and how they provide holistic healing at their clinic.

Why is Ayurveda Called a Root Cause Treatment?

Ayurveda is the ancient method of medical healing that focuses on the root cause of a condition. This form of medicine doesn't just cure your symptoms, it heals the areas of your body which are causing your symptoms. When you visit an experienced Ayurvedic practitioner, they'll explain how Ayurvedic treatments will target the chief causes of your medical condition.

Why Do Herbs Have No Major Side Effects?

Ayurvedic medicines are produced from completely natural herbs. There are no synthesized chemicals added to this kind of medicine, which therefore reduces the chances of negative side effects. Similarly, each treatment is highly customized based upon the observation of the symptoms and other medical tests.

How Do Herbs Help to Cure Diseases?

Herbs are well-known for their natural healing properties, and Ayurvedic medicines use the extracts of these herbs to cure different diseases in a variety of ways. Various herbs have healing properties that help restore balance within the body, the mind, and the soul, too.

What Are the Basic Principles of Ayurvedic Medicine?

Ayurveda recognizes 3 primary energies that form the 5 elements seen in the universe. These basic energies are vata, pitta, and kapha. They are seen within the processes of growth, maintenance, and decay, and their actions are known as anabolism, metabolism, and catabolism.

What is a Pulse Reading, and How is it Used in Ayurvedic Practice?

A pulse reading is a practice where the practitioner feels your pulse to detect vibrations that represent the metabolic processes going on within the physical body. These vibrations are related to the basic energies within the body. When trained well, Ayurvedic practitioners can read the pulse, and they can determine which area of your body is imbalanced and accordingly create a cure for you.

Is Ayurveda Really Efficient for Chronic Illnesses?

There are many chronic illnesses that Ayurveda has effectively helped, but the results of these treatments are often slow. Ayurveda offers treatments for autoimmune disorders, genital herpes, diabetes, alopecia, and other diseases as well.

The Importance of Evaluation & the Treatment of Imbalances

Ayurveda utilizes various techniques for the assessment of an individual's health. The Ayurveda practitioner considers and evaluates the key signs and symptoms of illness, especially with regards to the origin and cause of the first imbalance. They'll also consider the individual's suitability for various types of treatments.

After this is done, the Ayurveda practitioner will arrive at a diagnosis through efforts which include the use of direct questioning, careful observation, and a physical exam, including inference. Basic techniques will be used, like taking the pulse, observing the tongue, looking closely at the eyes and the body's form, and even listening to the tonality of the voice during the overall assessment.

Always Use a Trained Ayurvedic Practitioner

If you were going to paint your house all by yourself, you might know the ins and outs of how it could be done. But chances are, there'll be a few mistakes here and there. So, with your health, you need to trust someone who knows what they're doing, and someone who has studied the practice very well and who is certified.

Don't place your health in untrustworthy hands, and always ask for certification before going ahead with any treatments or tests, and in this way, you'll have peace of mind. After all, your health truly is your biggest asset. *Right?* Right.

Truly Knowing the Theory of Macrocosm/Microcosm & the Doshas

Punchamahabhutic concepts, when combined with the understanding of microcosm and macrocosm, provide colorful analogies about the doshas. Within the macrocosm/microcosm theory is the understanding that there's a continual interaction going on between the internal and external environment (or universe).

It can be understood as the macrocosm being governed by cosmic forces and the microcosm being governed by the principles of vata, pitta and kapha. And according to Ayurvedic principles, the first requirement for healing oneself (or others), is a clear understanding of the 3 dosha types. Studying each dosha is important, especially if the individual wants to become an Ayurvedic practitioner or even just to know themselves better.

The Interplay of the Doshas

The interplay of the 3 doshas gives the body both life and movement. The doshas are simultaneously the '3 blisses' and the '3 troubles.' And this is because, when they're balanced, they sustain the body, but when they're imbalanced they harm the body.

Each dosha has 3 states:

1. Vrddhi (or the state of aggravation)
2. Kesaya (or the state of diminution)
3. Samiya (or the state of equilibrium)

Applying the Tri-dosha Theory

The Tri-dosha theory applies to food, plants, and other elements of the environment:

For example, the dosha vata is found in the lower region of the human body. It's located below the navel, urinary, bladder, pelvic region, thighs, legs, and bones.

For pitta, it's located in the middle part between the navel and chest, and more exactly in the small intestine, stomach, sweat, lymph, and blood.

For kapha, it's in the upper part where the thorax, head, neck, joints, and fat tissues are located.

Vata is more dominant in older age, and in the evenings. Pitta dominates during adulthood, and during midday. Kapha dominates during youth and in the early morning.

The Ecological Aspects of Punchamahabhuta

According to the principles of punchamahabhuta, every living thing is connected. Living in balance and harmony with other beings is truly essential in terms of Ayurveda and its principles.

The plant kingdom gives oxygen, and from nature we get wood (for heat, building, paper, and more). It also gives us fibers for cloth, and from the animals we get manure to keep the soil fertile, as well as a plethora of other beneficial uses.

Ayurvedic models are purposely built to show the parallel growth patterns of various species, like the human fetus and a tree seed, for example.

The stages of growth are said to be the same, despite their obvious differences:

1. Expansion
2. Unidirectional growth
3. Conversion
4. Liquefaction
5. New growth

Living in Harmony with Other Creatures of the Earth

Most ancient people hold a deep respect for animals. And by observing animals, yogis and yoginis (practitioners of yoga) developed many yogic asanas (postures).

It's also true that Ayurvedic pharmacology was much enhanced by observing animals who recognized the medicinal qualities of plants, especially birds, like eagles and falcons. Other helpful and studied animals include goats, porcupines, oxen, serpents, and sheep.

The ecological and holistic aspects of Ayurveda are uniquely woven into the very definition of this system of healthcare. It's therefore difficult to extract what's not ecological about Ayurveda. It works and builds upon the ideal of connectedness, where the earth is the home of all living things.

The wellbeing of the earth is the wellbeing of all her inhabitants, and the destruction of the earth is the destruction of all her inhabitants. It's also important to note: all Ayurvedic medicines are derived directly from the earth, and only some are changed chemically.

The Weather & It's Constituents Are Part of Ayurveda, Too

Weather and climate winds, moonshine, sunshine, darkness, cold, heat, rain, day, night, fortnight, months, solstices, and seasons, well, these all play a part in the accumulation, augmentation, pacification, and reduction within the bodily processes and individual's state of being.

184

The most interesting part is the ecological aspects of Ayurveda, which include the connection between the seasonal changes *and* the activities of human beings. When the seasons move, earth-based cultures adjust to these changes as best as possible. And it can be paralleled with how some types of bears hibernate during the wintertime or that squirrels gather and store nuts before winter. And even some birds migrate to warmer climates for the winter season, too.

Ayurveda is an Ecologically Based, Ancient Principle, & Theory-Based Practice

We have come to the conclusion of the exploration of one system of holistic medicine, and so we can truly grasp that Ayurvedic healthcare concentrates on the health and wellbeing of the individual as a whole, and also as a member within society.

We have learned that most medicines and remedies are relatively low priced and affordable, and based upon food and herbs as pharmacological necessities. There are up to 8000+ recipes for the distinct preparation of different medicines within Ayurveda. The pharmacological aspects of Ayurveda are well developed and have true efficacy, too. Generally speaking, there aren't unpleasant side effects experienced when a trained Vaidya is recommending treatment to their client, either.

Ayurvedic methods of diagnosis are both simple and non-invasive. The understanding of a disease reflects the interactions between both the mind and body of the individual in question. In Ayurveda, the emphasis is placed upon positive health and the sustaining of prevention of disease. A wholesome diet and recommended daily regimen assist in overall health promotion, too.

Ayurveda is close to nature in the sense that it's an ecological system of healthcare which takes pride in treating every individual uniquely. It goes hand in hand with yoga, as Ayurveda was developed to build up the body, and yoga was designed to develop the spirit (or soul) of the individual.

Ayurveda places the utmost importance upon the constitution or resting state of the individual. The choices and dosage of medicines are dependent upon dosha and upon the surrounding environmental conditions, and so, the treatment plans are individualized to people's unique needs, a poignant difference from the Westernized system of healthcare, in fact. Most Ayurvedic practitioners and clients maintain an open attitude to other systems of medicine, however.

And so, dietary habits, remedies, and healthful daily routines may vary from locality to locality, but their principles remain the same. That is, to: observe harmonious relationships in all areas of life, and within nature, too.

Ayurveda may be practiced in a self-sufficient manner in any climate and may also allow the individual to decrease their dependence on modern (Western) experts and on drug companies.

An Interesting Phenomenon of Thought

As a last note, dhatus are the 7 basic and vital tissues or constructing elements. Malas are known as the waste products.

Interestingly, ether may be difficult to understand for those not trained in Indian science. But the ether is said to be "space," "emptiness," "vacuousness," and "distance." Sub-atomically, it's the 'nothingness' where the electron rotates around the atom. In modern chemistry, it's widely understood that matter is mostly composed of nothing. And so, this is the ancient Indian concept of akash, where nothingness is a part of all matter.

Akash is not endowed with any kind of action. It's said to be one of the biggest dimensions possible and the common receptacle of all things within the universe. It's shapeless. Within the field of quantum mechanics, akash is equivalent to the Western medical field and its drug companies. A common thought of Ayurvedic practitioners, where in contrast, Ayurveda would be the opposite, or "plentifulness." Of course, each individual can decide for themselves, where their belief system resides.

References:

China's new quality control, functional foods and nutraceuticals, 2003. http://www.ffnuag.com/ASP/377/

Cheng JT. Review: drug therapy in Chinese traditional medicine. J Clin Pharmacol. 2000;40:445–50. [PubMed] [Google Scholar]

Draft guidelines: Guidance for Industry—Botanical drug products—United States Food, Drug Administration—CDER. 2000. Available at http://www.fda.gov/cder/guidance/4592fnl.htm.

EMEA Guidance on Herbal Products The European Agency for the Evaluation of Medicinal Products, London, 2001. Available at www.emea.eu.int/pdfs/human/qwp/281900en.pdf.

Farnsworth NR. Relative safety of herbal medicines. Herbalgram. 1993;29:36A-H. [Google Scholar]

Gavaghan H. Koop may set up new center for alternative medicine. Nature. 1994;370:591. [PubMed] [Google Scholar]

Hankey A. CAM modalities can stimulate advances in theoretical biology. Evid Based Complement Alternat Med. 2005;2:5–12. [PMC free article] [PubMed] [Google Scholar]

Lad V. Ayurveda: The Science of Self-Healing. Wilmot: Lotus Press; 1985. The human constitution; pp. 26–36. [Google Scholar]

Marccus DM, Grollman AP. Botanical medicines—the need for new regulations. New Engl J Med. 2002;347:2073–6. [PubMed] [Google Scholar]

Mukherjee PK. Quality Control Herbal Drugs. New Delhi: Business Horizons; 2002. Herbal drugs-toxicity and regulations; pp. 39–87. [Google Scholar]

Quality Control Guidelines for Medicinal Plant Materials. Geneva: World Health Organization; 1998. Available at http://www.who.int/medicines/library/trm/medicinalplants/qualitycontrolmeth.pdf. [Google Scholar]

Sharma DC. India raises standards for traditional drugs. Lancet. 2000;356:231. [PubMed] [Google Scholar]

Warude D, Patwardhan B. Botanicals: quality and regulatory issues. J Sci Ind Res. 2005;64:83–92. [Google Scholar]

Suggested Reading:

Ayurvedic Healing 2nd Edition - *David Frawley*

Ayurveda: Life, Health & Longevity - *Robert E. Svoboda*

Ayurveda: The Science of Self-Healing - *Vasant Lad*

The Book of Ayurveda: A Holistic Approach to Health & Longevity - *Judith H. Morrison*